OTHER BOOKS IN THE 10 BEST QUESTIONS™ SERIES
BY DEDE BONNER, PH.D.

The 10 Best Questions™ for Surviving Breast Cancer
The 10 Best Questions™ for Living with Alzheimer's

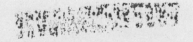

The 10 Best
QUESTIONS™

for *Recovering from a Heart Attack*

The Script You Need
to Take Control of Your Health

DEDE BONNER, PH.D.

FOREWORD BY DR. VICKI RACKNER

A FIRESIDE BOOK
PUBLISHED BY SIMON & SCHUSTER
NEW YORK LONDON TORONTO SYDNEY

This book is dedicated to my mother,
Jane J. Anderson, whose heart attack ten years ago
inspired me to ask more questions.

Fireside
A Division of Simon & Schuster, Inc.
1230 Avenue of the Americas
New York, NY 10020

First Fireside trade paperback edition May 2009

FIRESIDE and colophon are registered trademarks of Simon & Schuster, Inc.

For information about special discounts for bulk purchases, please contact Simon & Schuster Special Sales at 1-800-456-6798 or business@simonandschuster.com.

Manufactured in the United States of America

10 9 8 7 6 5 4 3 2 1

Library of Congress Cataloging-in-Publication Data

Bonner, Dede.
    The 10 best questions for recovering from a heart attack: the script you need to take control of your health / by Dede Bonner.
        p. cm.
    "A Fireside Book."
    Includes index.
1. Myocardial infarction—Popular works. I. Title. II. Title.
    RC685.I6B655 2009   2008043228
    616.1'237—dc22
ISBN-13: 978-1-4165-6052-4
ISBN-10:   1-4165-6052-1

Acknowledgments

I would like to thank the following people who made this book possible: my devoted husband, Randy Bonner; my loving mother, Jane Anderson; my brilliant editor at Simon & Schuster, Michelle Howry; my literary agent, Paul Fedorko of the Trident Media Group; former Simon & Schuster CEO, Jack Romanos; editor-in-chief of Touchstone Fireside, Trish Todd; and my attorney, Lisa E. Davis, of Frankfurt Kurnit Klein & Selz, PC; all of whom believed in me and in my vision for the 10 Best Questions™ series. A special thanks also to Dr. Caela Farren for being there for me.

I'd like to thank the experts I interviewed for this book for graciously sharing their time and expertise and for reviewing my drafts, especially Dr. Vicki Rackner for her foreword, and Kathy Berra, MSN, of Stanford University, for her comprehensive medical review.

Thanks to my university colleagues, Dr. John P. Fry, Dr. Donald G. Roberts, and Dr. Virginia Bianco-Mathis of Marymount University in Arlington, Virginia; Dr. Cynthia Roman and Dr.

Elizabeth B. Davis of The George Washington University in Washington, D.C.; and Dr. Margaret Nowak, Dr. Robert Evans, and Dr. Alison Preston, of Curtin University of Technology in Perth, Western Australia.

Lastly, I want to thank all of my graduate business students in the United States and Australia for their enthusiasm, research efforts, and questions. I'd especially like to thank the following students who researched related topics as their class projects and the experts they interviewed.

From Curtin University of Technology in Perth, Western Australia: Muna Abdullah Al-Raisi, Lisa Best, Felicite Black, Russell Byrne, Linda Deutsch, Craig D'Souza, Stephen Dunstan, John Gourlay, Cheryl Hayward, Judy Hargrave, Mark Hort, Ashley Hunt, Tanya Jardine, Brad Kelly, Mark Latham, Ronellie Lenon, Erika Lozano, Michelle Murray, Carmen Ng, Sharin Ruba, Cheree Schneider, Balwant Singh, John Stopp, Jennifer Talbot, Alan Thornton, Anne VanDenElzen, John Wareing, and Peter Westlund.

From Marymount University in Arlington, Virginia: Jaime Boyer, Arend Fish, Kelly Foster, Jennifer Hanley, Shannon Hiltner, Michelle Ray, and George Straubs.

Contents

Foreword

---

by Vicki Rackner, MD

Talk about a wake-up call! You most likely remember the precise moment your doctor told you that your heart was less than perfectly healthy. Questions may have flooded your mind. Will I need an operation? How do I get the very best medical care possible? Is there hope for me, given my family history?

As you peel back the layers of questions, you find one at the very core. *Can I really make a difference in my heart health?*

The good news is that you can influence the quality of your medical care. Your actions can influence the health of your heart. And you can overcome an ominous family history and recover from heart disease.

That's why I'm so glad you picked up this book. When you ask the right questions, you are directed to the right actions that can make a difference in the way your heart works. No matter how grim the situation seems—even if you're pounds from your target weight, or your idea of exercise is getting off the couch to turn off the TV, or you've started smoking (again!)—today you can decide to ask some different questions, make some different choices, and move your heart in the direction of health rather than disease.

The overall health of your heart is like a scorecard that tallies all of the choices you make each and every day. At any point you can turn this game around. Even choices that seem unrelated, like whether you reach out when you're lonely, contribute to the way your heart works.

If you think that although there might be hope for other people, there is none for you because everyone in your family dies young from heart disease, please think again. Your genes are not your destiny. Yes, you have a less favorable scorecard than you would have if you came from a different family, which makes your day-to-day choices even more important.

If you're a woman and think that you need to worry about your breasts but not your heart, think again. Cardiovascular disease is the number one killer of American women.

If you think that being an empowered patient ends after selecting the most prestigious medical center, please think again. It's important for all patients (even those being treated by the very best medical professionals) to take an active hand in their own health. Even the best-intentioned doctors and nurses make mistakes. Your ability to ask the right questions can literally save your life.

If your wake-up call came months ago, you might have slipped back into your old habits. A year after a heart attack, 60 percent of patients have stopped taking their medicine—medicine that studies definitively show will decrease the risk of a second heart attack. It's crucial that you stay in close contact with your doctor and stay on your heart-healthy program.

Heart health is everyone's business. The ability to ask good questions and make good choices can literally be the difference between life and death. It's also a legacy you pass on to your children.

In my experience of treating tens of thousands of patients, I notice patterns. Quite often, patients with heart disease are the people in the family everyone turns to for support and nurturing. They're the heart of the family. Many put the needs of others first and then get to their own needs if and when time and energy allow.

My hope for you is that when you listen to your heart's wake-up call, you hear it's time for you to nourish yourself first. Just as the doctors' procedures and medications can open the door to a healthier heart, so, too, you can open the way to a healthier way of working with your doctors and making better day-to-day choices. The right questions are like the cardiologist's balloon that opens up blocked blood vessels to the heart. By asking the right questions, you may prevent the need for the services of that invasive cardiologist. You can and will direct your heart toward better health.

Vicki Rackner, MD, is a board-certified surgeon who left the operating room to help patients, patients' families, and caregivers partner more effectively with their doctors through her company, Medical Bridges. She is also an author, speaker, and consultant, including coauthor of a Chicken Soup for the Soul: Healthy Living Series *book and several patient self-help books. Her Web site is www.medicalbridges.com.*

Introduction

The most important questions are often the ones you didn't know to ask. Even the best doctors in the world can't give you the right answers unless you ask them the right questions first.

But how do you know what the right questions are? "Ask your doctor." You've heard it a million times, but do you *really* know what to ask? What if you don't know very much about heart disease, feel intimidated by your doctor's expertise, or simply feel overwhelmed by your diagnosis or the diagnosis of a loved one?

More than ten years ago when my mother suffered a major heart attack, I felt overwhelmed. As I nervously watched her vital sign monitors bounce around, it occurred to me that I didn't know what to ask the doctors about her condition. In that moment of total helplessness, the only thing I had was questions. But I just didn't know what to ask.

I vowed to learn how to ask better questions. When I started taking my mom to her follow-up doctor appointments, I spent time researching her medical options and planning questions for her doctor. I wanted to be a well-informed consumer for her sake so that I could make sure she was getting the very best care possible.

This experience sparked my interest in questioning skills. As I read about questions, I was surprised to learn how little attention most people pay to them. It seems that our society is so focused on solutions and answers that we rarely stop to consider the quality of our questions.

I started teaching questioning skills as part of my graduate-level business classes in Washington, D.C., and Perth, Australia. My students liked it so much that I developed the concept of "The 10 Best Questions" as a way for them to learn questioning skills, team dynamics, and research skills all at once. Since 2003, I've taught hundreds of students who have interviewed thousands of experts. For example, my students have researched what to ask when you buy a house, get married, adopt a dog, hire a financial planner, change careers, invest in stocks, retire, plan a wedding, talk to your teenagers, choose a university, and for great sex.

To learn their secrets, I conducted a series of interviews with top question askers. Helen Thomas, the legendary White House reporter, is famous for her press conference questions to every president since John F. Kennedy. She told me, "Before a news conference I would think, What's the best question to ask? I have the courage of ignorance in my questions. I always get nervous, figuring out what to ask a president. But I believe you have to be curious and keep asking why."

Dorothy Leeds, who has authored nine books on questioning skills, told me, "Everything in my life has come about from asking questions, every major change. It's amazing how questions can enrich your life, both from a career and personal standpoint."

Peter Block, an international management consultant and the author of the book *The Answer to How Is Yes,* said, "There's a deeper meaning to asking questions. It's a stance you take in the world, a desire to make contact and get connected."

I talked with many professional interviewers like Susan Sikora, a TV talk show host in San Francisco; Debbie Nigro, a New York radio host; and Richard Koonce, a journalist and consultant in Brookline, Massachusetts. Each responded with a version of, "You are only as good as the questions you ask." Since then, I've focused my consulting work on helping CEOs and organizations develop their own Best Questions.

For the information specific to this book, I interviewed two former U.S. surgeons general and the president of the American Heart Association. I also interviewed prominent experts in cardiology, heart surgery, cardiac rehabilitation, nutrition, exercise, women's cardiac issues, preventive heart health, stress, fitness, special populations, smoking and alcohol cessation, and personal and family relationships.

So, what are the traits of the best question askers? They are smart, curious, and fearless, yet humble enough to learn from someone else. They value listening and inquiry. Great question askers see every person they meet as a walking encyclopedia of valuable information just waiting to be unlocked by the right questions. And finally, as Albert Einstein once said, "The difference between me and everyone else is my ability to ask the right questions."

The 10 Best Questions in this book won't make you an instant Einstein. And as the Question Doctor, I certainly don't claim any Einstein-like brilliance. I believe that a good mind knows the right answers, but a great mind knows the right questions. Now that great mind is yours. This book is for "smarties," not dummies.

Each list of The 10 Best Questions is derived from as many as nine hundred questions from hundreds of sources, including books, journals, worldwide print media, Web sites, and expert interviews. A Best Question has to really earn its title of "Best." I've also included the "best answers" that my experts and research provided so that you'll know when you are hearing the full story. The information in this book should not replace medical guidance or professional counseling.

There is one more question per chapter that I call "The Magic Question™." A Magic Question is that one great question that even smart people rarely think to ask—a gut-level question you usually think of when it's too late.

In writing this book, I've taken a practical and holistic approach to heart disease to make you an empowered patient. I want to help with your key decisions, choices, and relationships by suggesting what you can ask your doctors, medical experts, partner, family, friends, and ultimately yourself after a heart attack or the diagnosis of heart disease.

Your lifetime prescription for good health is to stay informed. As former surgeon general Dr. C. Everett Koop told me in an interview, "There's nothing that will lead to better medical care than a knowledgeable patient."

The 10 Best Questions in this book give you the actual script in hand for each major conversation and decision you are facing. Be sure to ask plenty of your own questions, too. Question guru Helen Thomas says, "There's no such thing as a bad question, only a lot of bad answers."

As the Question Doctor, I sincerely hope that this book will give you the strength, comfort, and knowledge you need to embrace a lifetime filled with good health—and lots of good questions.

through interruptions. If your doctor interrupts you before you make your point, try saying, "I'd like to finish," or, "Can we come back to my concerns later?"

This book is primarily for people who have already had a heart attack, but it will also be valuable if you've been diagnosed with heart disease. The Best Questions in the first chapter suggest what to ask your doctor when you or your loved one is first recovering from a heart attack. Chapter 2 guides you in what to ask about heart disease whether or not you've had a heart attack. Use chapters 3 and 4 to find a great doctor, then chapters 5 and 6 to fully understand your diagnostic tests, medical procedures, and for a second opinion. Take chapter 7 with you to the doctor's office when you are going for follow-up appointments to discuss your risk factors. Chapter 8 covers special concerns for women with heart problems.

This book isn't necessarily meant to be read from cover to cover but rather to be grabbed and consulted for each crossroad and conversation in your journey back to a healthier heart. Remember that even the best doctors in the world can't give you the right answers if you don't ask the right questions.

PART I

Talking with Your Doctor

Two common concerns expressed by people who have survived a heart attack or have been diagnosed with heart disease are fear of the unknown and fear of not communicating well with their doctors. Your doctors can help you make decisions, but you have to ask the right questions first.

Many people are intimidated by their doctors' knowledge and are reluctant to ask them questions. Former acting U.S. surgeon general rear admiral Dr. Kenneth P. Moritsugu comments, "For the older generation, the relationship is that the doctor knows everything and you just accept what the doctor has to say."

But patient–physician relationships are changing. The president of the American Heart Association, Dr. Timothy J. Gardner, says, "A patient who has had a cardiac event or a major scare is very vulnerable and not necessarily wanting to challenge the doctor regarding options, especially if the doctor seems fairly certain about one course or another. But I think empowerment of the patient is something we really need to stress, not in a disagreeable way but so that patients can truly understand all their medical options."

Use this book to help you. This is no time to be shy, worry about hurting the doctor's feelings, or be secretly afraid that he or she may not "like you" if you ask questions. There's no reason to be aggressive in asking your questions, but be firm with your doctor that you expect answers.

To be heard, you may need to repeat your questions or concerns. According to a 1999 study published in *JAMA: The Journal of the American Medical Association,* when patients are trying to talk, doctors typically interrupt after just twenty-three seconds. Persist

CHAPTER 1: THE 10 BEST QUESTIONS

About Your Heart Attack

As for me, except for an occasional heart attack, I feel as
young as I ever did.

—Robert Benchley, American humorist

Heart disease can sneak up on you in the prime of life.
Like a lion stalking its prey, it moves silently into your
heart's arteries and waits to pounce as a heart attack or
chest pains (angina). Most people don't realize they have heart disease until they develop symptoms, chest discomfort, have pain,
shortness of breath, or have a heart attack.

You are not alone. In the United States, heart disease is the
number one killer of both men and women. It takes another life
every thirty-four seconds. Every year, more than 1.5 million people
in the United States have a heart attack. About four hundred to five
hundred thousand of them die. Half of the deaths occur before
reaching the hospital.

A heart attack happens when the blood flow to a section of your
heart muscle becomes completely blocked. If the flow of blood
isn't restored quickly, the heart becomes starved for oxygen, is
damaged, and begins to die. The medical terms for a heart attack
are **myocardial infarction, coronary thrombosis,** and **coronary
occlusion.**

The main culprit in heart attacks is **coronary artery disease**
(also called **CAD**), which results when a fatty material called
plaque builds up over many years on the inside walls of your coronary arteries (the arteries that supply blood and oxygen to your
heart). An area of plaque can rupture suddenly, causing a blood clot

---

THE QUESTION DOCTOR SAYS:

Ask your doctor for the basics now. You can learn more about your heart disease and how to manage it during follow-up conversations or office visits with your doctor.

If possible, use a notepad or recording device to capture the doctor's answers. There may be a lot of information coming at you just as you are on the verge of an emotional meltdown. Ask a family member or a nurse to take notes for you.

There is nothing more comforting or empowering than being a well-informed patient. Don't be afraid to ask other questions or for the doctor to repeat anything you don't understand.

---

to form on the surface of the plaque. If the clot becomes large enough, it can block the flow of oxygen-rich blood to the heart.

The diagnosis of a heart attack is made from your symptoms, the electrocardiogram, and blood tests taken during your initial evaluation. This chapter's Best Questions assume that you've already had a heart attack and are now well enough to have a conversation with your doctor. A loved one or a nurse can also ask these Best Questions on your behalf.

〉〉〉THE 10 BEST QUESTIONS
About Your Heart Attack

1. Did I have a heart attack? How do you know for sure?

The first step in diagnosing a heart attack is to be suspicious that one has occurred, especially if you didn't have the classic crushing chest pains or other typical symptoms. About one-third of all heart attacks lack dramatic symptoms, especially for women.

Your medical team is likely to be fairly certain. Tests can quickly confirm a heart attack, so emergency treatments can be started immediately to restore blood flow and minimize heart damage.

An **electrocardiogram (ECG or EKG)** records the electrical abnormalities typical of a heart attack and can identify the areas of the heart muscle that were deprived of oxygen and damaged. Blood tests measure the cardiac enzymes (**creatine phosphoki-nase** or **CPK,** special subfractions of CPK, and **troponin**) that are typically elevated in the blood several hours after a heart attack. A series of blood tests during the first twenty-four hours confirms the heart attack and the amount of heart muscle that has died.

A heart attack is very different from **cardiac arrest** or **sudden cardiac death.** A blockage stops blood flow during a heart attack, as compared to cardiac arrest, when the heart suddenly stops beating due to abnormal or irregular heart rhythms (called **ventricular arrhythmias**).

2. Why did I have this heart attack? What caused it?

The definition of a heart attack is the death of heart muscle due to the sudden blockage of a coronary artery by a ruptured blood vessel that causes a blood clot. **Coronary arteries** are the blood vessels that supply blood and oxygen to the heart.

A blockage causes injury to the heart muscle, chest pain, and the feeling of chest pressure or other symptoms. These other symptoms include sensations like indigestion, burning, a tightness or heaviness, feeling like a band or belt is tightening across your chest, jaw discomfort, back pain, numbness in your arms, a shortness of breath, or unusual fatigue.

Blockages are caused by plaque buildup in a process called **atherosclerosis.** Atherosclerosis has no symptoms, which is why heart attacks often surprise their victims and are called "silent killers." Symptoms from atherosclerosis generally occur only after the blockage is greater than 70 percent. But many heart attacks are caused by blockages of less than 50 percent that rupture. When this happens, the result is a blood clot in the artery that causes a complete blockage and results in a heart attack.

3. How much heart damage is there? Where is the damage located? Is my heart permanently damaged?

Time spent is heart muscle lost. The longer it took to get medical attention after the onset of your heart attack, the more heart damage there is. The heart muscle that has lost blood supply begins to die. The amount of damage depends on the size of the affected area and the time between onset and treatment.

If the blood flow is not restored within a few minutes, the affected heart muscle cells can suffer permanent damage or die. Irreversible death of the heart muscle begins within twenty to forty minutes from onset. But the heart is very tough and can keep working even if a part of it has died. The heart heals itself by forming scar tissue.

Future complications depend in part on the location of the damage (either the right or left **ventricles,** which are the lower heart chambers). Your outcome is worse if the heart attack caused significant damage to the heart muscle and resulted in heart failure. Heart failure can be treated with medications (see chapter 9) and lifestyle changes (see part 3). Ask your doctor to explain more.

In addition, heart muscle damage can result in damage to the electrical signaling system that tells the heart to contract. Some people need a pacemaker to correct this function of the heart muscle.

4. What is my ejection fraction?

The **ejection fraction** is a comparison of the quantity of blood ejected from the heart's left ventricle during its contraction phase with the quantity of blood remaining at the end of the left ventricle's relaxation phase. A normal ejection fraction reading is between 60 and 70 percent.

If the heart muscle is damaged during a heart attack, it has an impaired ability to eject blood. This reduces the ejection fraction, which can result in heart failure.

The ejection fraction is one of the most important predictors of your **prognosis** (long-term health outlook). People with a significantly reduced ejection fraction typically have a poorer prognosis. However, with time to heal and the use of medications for heart failure, your heart can improve its ability to pump blood.

5. Which tests, treatments, and medications was I given?

If you had a heart attack, you probably were in the hospital's **intensive care unit (ICU)** or **coronary care unit (CCU)** and may have needed several days in the hospital to recover. You probably received several different tests and may have had a procedure called **angioplasty** or **coronary artery stenting** to open blocked coronary arteries. Some people need emergency **coronary artery bypass surgery (CABG)**. See chapter 10.

You most likely received oxygen and were hooked up to an ECG machine to monitor your heartbeat. You may have received blood thinners, aspirin, and other medicines.

Find out the details, write them down, and request that copies of your medical records be sent to your family doctor.

6. Please explain my treatment options for interventions, surgeries, or medications. Which ones do you recommend and why?

Dr. Paul Kligfield, a medical director at New York's Cardiac Health Center, says, "Some patients tell their doctors, 'If I have a heart attack, *you* take care of it.' But the patient really needs to monitor his own treatment, risks, side effects, and problems. Patients are the ones with the disease, not the doctors, so they need to be actively involved."

Another important question is, "What happens if I choose to do nothing?" Choosing to do nothing must be a conscious decision reached by you with your doctor, not a denial of your heart attack or diagnosis. It's only natural to want to pretend it never happened. However, for most patients after a heart attack or with unstable, progressive heart disease, medical or interventional treatment and lifestyle changes will reduce the risk of additional cardiac events.

Also ask, "How long do I have to make decisions about treatments?" Depending on your heart's damage and disease and the amount of atherosclerosis in your arteries, you may have more time than you think for some clearheaded thinking and research.

Ask (especially if you've had major heart damage), "Do I need a **pacemaker** or an implantable **internal defibrillator?**" These are implanted devices that help to regulate your heart's rhythm or prevent cardiac arrest. See chapter 10.

Be careful to follow your doctor's recommendations. Many heart attack survivors are vulnerable to complications, especially soon after their cardiac event.

7. What can I do to help prevent another heart attack?

Your doctor will discuss risk factors and possible medications, surgery, or procedures. There are actions that your doctor will take (like performing surgery or prescribing medicine) as well as risk factors out of your control (age, gender, etc.).

But the point of this question is to learn what actions *you* can take personally and proactively to heal your broken heart. Think of this question as the beginning of a lifelong conversation about the lifestyle changes you are willing to make to help yourself and your heart. See part three of this book.

Medical experts unanimously agree that the most important things you can do to prevent another heart attack are the following:

- Quit smoking.
- Get more physical activity.
- Eat heart-healthy foods.
- Maintain a normal weight.
- Go to a cardiac rehabilitation program.
- Take medications.

8. Which lifestyle changes are the most important and will make me feel better?

Even if you were dealt a bad hand due to a family history of heart disease, you can fight back by controlling what you eat and your physical activity. Better lifestyle habits can dramatically reduce your risk for another heart attack and even reverse heart disease. Hearing this from your doctor is your most important first step to inspire you to make changes during your recovery.

Of course, for most people these changes are much easier said than done, especially if you belong to the couch potato club. This is why starting and sticking with a cardiac rehabilitation program is vital. Your goal is to improve your lifelong health habits.

9. Will you give me a referral for a cardiac rehabilitation program? How soon can I start?

If you are talking with your cardiologist, ask for a referral for a cardiac rehabilitation program. If you are talking with a doctor who you aren't likely to see again, hold on to this question until you are with your cardiologist or primary care physician.

See chapter 12 to understand why this is a Best Question, especially if you are older, a woman, or a person of color.

10. Considering my age and physical condition, how long will my recovery take? When can I resume my normal activities?

You'll want to know when you can start driving, working, and exercising. Ask again if you aren't sure or if the doctor gives you a vague answer.

Also ask these other important questions:

- Are there any activities I should avoid altogether? If so, for how long?
- Will my chest pains, weakness, and other symptoms go away?
- When can I safely have sex again?
- Are my feelings (depression, sadness, etc.) normal?
- How normal a life can I expect now?
- Do I need someone to care for me when I first get home from the hospital?
- When should I call you if I think I'm having symptoms?
- Do I need nitroglycerine tablets?

❯ The Magic Question

What are the warning signs of another heart attack? What should I do?

Knowing these warning signs can save your life.

A heart attack is a medical emergency. If you have the symptoms of a heart attack, seek immediate medical help by calling 911, even if you aren't sure. *Don't wait more than five minutes.*

Some heart attacks are sudden and intense, but most heart attacks start slowly with only mild pain initially. This is why some people wait too long to get help. Here are the warning signs:

- Chest, neck, jaw, back, or arm pain
- Upper body discomfort
- Heaviness in your chest

- Squeezing or a tight band around your chest
- Shortness of breath
- Cold sweat
- Nausea or vomiting
- Lightheadedness

Kathy Berra, MSN, the clinical director of Stanford University's Heart Network, simplifies the list of "triggers" for heart symptoms or chest pains. She says, "Remember the four E's: exercise, exertion, exposure to cold, and eating a large meal. If you have any warning signs plus one of the four E's, be sure to let your doctor know immediately. If the symptoms don't go away with rest, call 911 and go to the nearest emergency room."

Women are more likely than men to experience the less common symptoms, like nausea or shortness of breath. See the American Heart Association's Web site (www.americanheart.org/presenter. jhtml?identifier=3053#Heart_Attack) for more information.

CONCLUSION

You can probably relate to management consultant Dr. Caela Farren's memory of her 2004 heart attack: "The background tape that kept running in my head was, 'This can't be happening to me!'"

The good news is that many heart attack survivors have an excellent prognosis thanks to modern advances. This is especially true if treatment is started within one hour of the onset of symptoms.

The most important factor in treating a heart attack is time. Dr. Spencer B. King, III, an executive director and the interim president of the Saint Joseph's Heart and Vascular Institute in Atlanta, says, "Time is muscle. Time is the key ingredient."

Dr. Timothy J. Gardner, president of the American Heart Association, concludes, "I want to make one thing very clear. There is

well-established evidence that the emergency treatment of heart attack patients with emergency or very rapid catheterization or clot-
busting drugs with catheters is the best treatment for patients with
acute heart attacks."

THE 10 BEST RESOURCES

American Heart Association. "Heart Attack Warning Signs." www.amer
icanheart.org/presenter.jhtml?identifier=3053.

American Heart Association. "Life After a Heart Attack." www.american
heart.org/presenter.jhtml?identifier=238.

American Heart Association. "What Is a Heart Attack?" www.american
heart.org/presenter.jhtml?identifier=3038238.

Arnot, Bob. *Seven Steps to Stop a Heart Attack.* New York: Simon & Schuster, 2005.

Cleveland Clinic. "Understanding Heart Failure." http://my.cleveland
clinic.org/heart/disorders/heartfailure/understanding_hf.aspx.

Kligfield, Paul. *The Cardiac Recovery Handbook: The Complete Guide to Life
After Heart Attack or Heart Surgery,* 2nd ed. Long Island City, NY: Hatherleigh Press, 2006.

Mayo Clinic. "Heart Attack." www.mayoclinic.com/health/heart-attack/
DS00094/DSECTION=1.

National Heart Lung and Blood Institute. "Act in Time to Heart Attack
Signs." www.nhlbi.nih.gov/actintime/index.htm.

WebMD. "Heart Failure." www.webmd.com/heart-disease/heart-failure/
default.htm.

Wikipedia. "Myocardial Infarction." http://en.wikipedia.org/wiki/Heart_
attack.

CHAPTER 2: THE 10 BEST QUESTIONS

About Your Heart Disease

> If you don't think every day is a good day, just try missing one.
>
> —Cavett Robert, American speaker

Many people have heart disease, but few understand it. According to the World Health Organization, heart disease killed at least seven million people worldwide in 2006 and is responsible for 30 percent of all deaths (about seven hundred thousand) in the United States every year.

If you have a recent diagnosis of heart disease or have had a heart attack, you face a whole new vocabulary of confusing and scary medical terms. Working with your doctor and asking good questions are your best defenses in fighting your heart disease and preventing your first or next heart attack.

Dr. Alfred Bove, the former chief of cardiology at Temple University Medical Center and the president of the American College of Cardiology, says, "Nowadays, it's really important for patients to know as much as they can about their illness. I'm an advocate of patient empowerment. The most important thing for people to understand is that they can understand their illness almost as much as the physician can. As a patient, you *can* talk to your doctor at the same level rather than having him talk down to you."

Ask your doctor the following Best Questions to understand your heart disease and your treatment options in more depth.

Note: As this book went to press, the results of a long-antici-pated major study were released by the American Heart Association. The study suggests that using **statins** (cholesterol reducing drugs) to treat the symptoms of inflammation, an oft-overlooked condition, may nearly halve people's risk of future heart attack, stroke, and heart-related death. Ask your doctor about having a **C-reactive protein (CRP) test** for inflammation and about taking statins.

THE QUESTION DOCTOR SAYS:

Don't ever hesitate to ask other questions that are not in this book. There truly are no dumb questions, especially for a diagnosis like heart disease. You have every right to know as much as you can about your heart's health. It's your body and you deserve having a well-educated mind inside of it.

⟩⟩⟩ THE 10 BEST QUESTIONS
About Your Heart Disease

1. What type of heart disease do I have? What is its medical name?

The term *heart disease* is used broadly here as an all-inclusive de-scription. Most people think there is only one type of heart disease, coronary artery disease (CAD), which is the buildup of fatty plaque on the inside of coronary arteries. This is by far the most common type and is the number one killer in the United States.

But there are numerous other diseases of the heart muscle, veins, arteries, and circulatory system that affect the heart. The most com-mon include:

- **Arrhythmia** (abnormal heart rhythms where the heart beats too fast, too slow, or is irregular). The most common type of arrhythmia is called **atrial fibrillation,** and it significantly increases the risk of having a stroke.

- **Angina** (chest pain or pressure occurs because the heart isn't getting enough blood).
- **Atherosclerotic heart disease** (slow buildup of a blockage in the arteries feeding oxygen to the heart).
- **Heart failure** (also called **congestive cardiac failure,** which is caused by structural or functional disorders).
- **Ischemia** (reduced blood to the heart which can result in angina).
- **Heart valve disease** (types include **valvular stenosis** and **valvular insufficiency**).
- **Congenital heart disease** (a heart defect present at birth).
- **Heart muscle inflammation** (called **cardiomyopathy,** with three main types: **dilated,** the most common type; **hypertrophic;** and **restrictive**).
- **Pericardial disease** (inflamed heart layers).
- **Vascular heart disease** (blood vessel disease).

2. What caused my heart disease?

The main type of heart disease, coronary artery disease, is caused by the slow buildup of fatty plaque on the inner walls of the heart's arteries in a process called **atherosclerosis.**

Other possible causes include past heart attacks (some people are unaware they've had one), abnormal heart valves, heart muscle disease (called **cardiomyopathy**), heart defects present at birth, severe lung disease, severe anemia (low red blood cell count), overactive thyroid (**hyperthyroidism**), and abnormal heart rhythms (called **arrhythmia** or **dysrhythmia**).

Your doctor may also address your risk factors. See Best Question 5 in this chapter.

3. What stage is my heart disease? Am I going to die soon?

In order to determine the best treatments for heart patients, doctors often assess the stage of a patient's heart failure using the New York Heart Association's four stages. These stages are simple and relate to everyday activities and your quality of life:

Class I (Mild). No symptoms and no limitations on activity.
Class II (Minimal). Mild symptoms with strenuous exercise.
Class III (Moderate). Marked symptoms prevent some activities.
Class IV (Severe). Noticeable symptoms, even at rest, and can be debilitating.

See more at the American Heart Association's Web site: www. americanheart.org/presenter.jhtml?identifier=1712.

Your doctor won't know your life expectancy with certainty, but most people ask this question anyway.

4. Please explain my treatment options. Do I need tests, procedures, surgeries, or medications? Which ones do you recommend and why?

Treatment of heart disease covers the spectrum, from getting more exercise to having a heart transplant. Ask your doctor to explain his or her recommendations and reasoning in detail. Be sure to ask this follow-up question: What pain or side effects can I expect from this treatment?

See also chapters 5 (tests and procedures), 9 (medications), and 10 (heart surgeries) for more specific questions.

5. What are my specific heart attack risk factors? Which ones can I do something about?

The risk factors that contribute to heart disease include:

- Smoking
- Elevated blood cholesterol

- Low HDL (good) cholesterol
- Physical inactivity
- Diabetes
- High blood pressure
- Being overweight
- Depression, stress, and social isolation
- Male gender
- Family history of heart attacks at an early age

See more questions about heart risks in chapter 7.

6. What lifestyle changes do I need to make? Which changes are the most important ones in my case?

Your doctor will probably talk about exercise, diet choices, weight management, and smoking cessation. By asking about your personal top priorities, you'll know what to tackle first.

Changing all your unhealthy lifelong habits at the same time is nearly impossible. The experts recommend setting smaller and more achievable goals. This is also important because some changes are interrelated, like quitting smoking and managing your weight. Here are smart follow-up questions:

- Which physical activities would I most benefit from?
- Do I need to lose weight? How much? Who or what can help me?
- What diet or program do you recommend?
- Where can I get help to quit smoking?

7. What else can I do to lower my chances of having a heart attack or stroke?

This question is very proactive and empowering. Ask for specific advice and recommendations. Your doctor may suggest certain genetic tests or other advanced blood tests to further clarify your risks. He may also mention working with a personal trainer to develop a regular exercise routine or finding a dietitian who can advise on healthier food choices.

8. Am I a good candidate for participating in a cardiac rehabilitation program? Why or why not?

If you have severe heart disease, ask your doctor if you are eligible for going to cardiac rehab, a supervised heart-healthy exercise and wellness program for heart attack survivors and some heart patients.

Harvard professor and cardiac rehab expert Dr. Daniel Forman says, "Ideally, cardiac rehab should happen before you have a heart attack if you have significant risk factors."

You'll have to get a doctor referral to participate. Cardiac rehab may really help you with making long-term lifestyle changes. But not all doctors automatically give referrals, especially if you haven't had a heart attack. See more in chapter 12.

9. Am I eligible and a good candidate for participating in a clinical trial? Why or why not?

Depending on the extent and type of heart disease, you may want to consider joining a clinical trial, which is a medical research project. Before you join a trial, ask lots of questions, especially about the study's sponsors, objectives, and how they protect patients' safety.

10. Where can I get more information about heart disease and how to prevent a heart attack?

Taking a proactive and education-focused approach will help you greatly as you start to make permanent heart-healthy lifestyle changes. Cardiologist Dr. Alfred Bove says, "The number one issue is that patients need to understand their disease. The expectations for me are that they will manage their own cardiovascular risk factors, not just take orders from me. Patients are like the managers of their own databases, but I'm managing five hundred databases [patient files]."

You can find extensive resources from the American Heart Association (www.americanheart.org), Cardiosmart (www.cardiosmart.org), and the resources in this book.

❯ The Magic Question

How can I tell the difference between angina or indigestion and a heart attack?

Indigestion can be a burning pain and angina is severe chest pain. Both may feel like a heart attack, but neither is likely to spread to other parts of the body. Pain shooting down your arms, especially if you don't normally suffer from indigestion or pain, may be the sign of a heart attack.

Ask your doctor to explain the warning signs of a heart attack and more details about how to tell the difference between angina or indigestion and a heart attack. Then tell your family members what your doctor said.

If you are in any doubt, don't hesitate to call 911 immediately, *not* your doctor's office. It's better to have a false alarm than not live to be embarrassed by it.

CONCLUSION

You may have realized you have heart disease only after waking up in the hospital's intensive care unit following a heart attack. Or your doctor may have diagnosed your heart disease based on tests and your symptoms or chest pains.

Being an empowered patient means being a key player on the medical team looking after your ailing heart. Develop the good habits of a healthy lifestyle and a questioning mind.

THE 10 BEST RESOURCES

American Heart Association. "Diagnosing Heart Disease." www.ameri canheart.org/presenter.jhtml?identifier=330.

American Heart Association. "Information for Patients." www.american heart.org/presenter.jhtml?identifier=3051963.

CardioSmart. "Manage My Condition." www.cardiosmart.org/Manage Condition.

Consumer Reports Health. "Shared Decision-Making: Working with Your Doctor." www.consumerreports.org. (Subscription required.)

Granato, Jerome E. *Living with Coronary Heart Disease: A Guide for Patients and Families.* Baltimore, MD: Johns Hopkins University Press, 2008.

Johns Hopkins Heart and Vascular Institute. "Johns Hopkins Heart Institute: Conditions." www.hopkinsheart.org/conditions-treatments/index .conditions.html.

Katzenstein, Larry, and Ileanna L. Pina. *Living with Heart Disease: Everything You Need to Know to Safeguard Your Health and Take Control of Your Life.* New York: Sterling Publishing, 2007.

MedlinePlus. "Heart Diseases." www.nlm.nih.gov/medlineplus/heart diseases.html.

National Heart, Lung, and Blood Institute. "Your Guide to Living Well with Heart Disease." www.nhlbi.nih.gov/health/public/heart/other/your_ guide/living_well.htm.

Superko, H. Robert, and Laura Tucker. *Before the Heart Attacks.* New York: Rodale Books, 2003.

CHAPTER 3: THE 10 BEST QUESTIONS

To Get Reliable Referrals for the Best Doctors and Surgeons

> A doctor who cannot take out your appendix properly will recommend you to a doctor who will be unable to remove your tonsils with success.
>
> —Ernest Hemingway

If you have had a heart attack or been diagnosed with heart disease, you may need a heart specialist, called a **cardiologist,** or a cardiac surgeon as the next step. Other people who have less serious heart disease may choose to continue with their regular doctor.

You may wish to consider establishing a long-term relationship with a cardiologist because heart disease is a chronic condition, which means you'll have it for the rest of your life. You want a cardiologist or cardiac surgeon who you can trust as a partner, a top doctor who will ensure the best quality of treatments and up-to-date knowledge on the latest heart drugs and research.

You can find a cardiologist or surgeon by asking for a referral from your primary care physician, family members, or friends. If you are like most people, the only questions you'll probably ask during this brief initial conversation are simple ones to get the new doctor's name, address, and phone number. Perhaps you'll ask, "Do you like this doctor?" or "Where is he located?" Most likely, you trust the person giving you the referral.

In blind faith, you call the prospective doctor's office and schedule the first appointment you can get. As you hang up, you feel a rush of relief because the doctor's receptionist wasn't from Mars and you could get in to see this new doctor quickly.

But you may have just jumped headfirst into potentially dangerous quicksand—and don't even know it. Here's why. It may not have occurred to you that you know virtually nothing about this new doctor. Okay, perhaps you did an Internet search, but you have already let your most important ally and information source slip away—the person who gave you this referral.

Stop and think about this for just a moment. Here you are on the brink of establishing a very important new relationship with the person who will ultimately hold your health and well-being in his hands. This doctor's judgment and experience will be absolutely critical at every step of the way.

You also can't assume that just because you've gotten a referral from your current doctor that this new doctor will automatically be great. Maybe you feel shy about questioning your current doctor closely about her referral, fearful you will somehow insult her judgment. Maybe you secretly worry your current doctor will think you are dumb or too aggressive if you ask more questions. Get over it. This is a very important referral and you have every right to know the qualifications of the doctors treating you.

There are hundreds of potential reasons behind the referral, ranging from the two of them being Friday night poker pals to being longtime partners in the operating room. The point is that you just don't know until you ask.

The following list of 10 Best Questions includes questions to ask in two scenarios. In the first situation, use questions 1 and 2 and the Magic Question when talking with someone with medical expertise.

In the second situation, you are getting the referral from current patients, friends, or family members—your peers. When talking with nonmedical people, ask all ten questions and the Magic Question. As you start, be sure to find out first if this prospective doctor honors your medical insurance and takes new patients.

Don't hesitate to ask questions. So much is at stake. Having a top doctor will make all the difference in your care. In chapter 4, you'll talk directly to this new doctor. But for now, don't skip this important preliminary step of getting a quality referral.

〉〉〉THE 10 BEST QUESTIONS
To Get Reliable Referrals for the
Best Doctors and Surgeons

1. Why are you recommending this doctor?

One of the best ways to judge a prospective doctor's quality is through the recommendation from another doctor. Most doctors are sincerely interested in the well-being of their patients and refer them to the doctors they believe offer the best care.

If you are asking a medical professional this question, listen for an answer that includes how impressive this specialist is in the field of cardiac research or surgery. Key phrases are "participated in clinical trials" and "presented papers at professional conferences." These are extra-effort activities that earn respect among medical peers. But don't stop there: Listen for clues about this prospective doctor's bedside manner as well as his superstar performance at last year's medical conference. However, as Phoenix cardiologist Dr. Rebecca Allison notes, "Some doctors who don't do research are still very good doctors."

Sometimes doctors fall into referral patterns of always recommending the same doctor down the hallway or a former college roommate. While this isn't necessarily a bad thing, it helps if you know this piece of background information.

If you are talking with other patients or friends, a good follow-up question is, "How did you originally find this doctor?" For example, if the person found this specialist without doing her homework, or even worse, from the Yellow Pages, take this person's diminished credibility into account as you assess her answers to your Best Questions below.

THE QUESTION DOCTOR SAYS:

Be sure to ask open-ended questions. For example, "How satisfied are you?" rather than "Are you satisfied?" A "how" question results in much more valuable information than a question that has a simple yes/no answer.

2. How well do you know him or her?

If you are asking a medical professional, you want to hear that this person has worked closely with the recommended doctor for a number of years. If you are seeking a second opinion, the doctors may not know each other as well, so listen for clues about the prospective doctor's reputation.

Don't assume that someone is a good cardiologist or surgeon just because your primary care doctor has referred you to him. You may learn they are only social friends and your doctor has little firsthand knowledge about his friend's real doctoring skills.

If you are asking a current patient, use this question to make sure her judgments aren't based on a short-lived or long-ago relationship.

3. How satisfied are you with this doctor? In your opinion, what are this doctor's strengths and areas that need improvement?

Depending on this person's degree of openness and willingness to talk, you may get all the details you need by simply asking how satisfied she is. Be sure to press gently for details on the areas that need improvement. Everyone has shortcomings. Use this question to decide if you can live with this doctor's particular deficiencies or quirks.

4. How well did this doctor communicate with you?

Listen for phrases like:

- I didn't feel rushed when I talked with him.
- He explained everything slowly and used words I could understand.
- He acted like he was really listening to me.
- He made me feel comfortable.
- I could finish my sentences without being interrupted.

5. How well has this doctor kept you informed and encouraged you to ask questions?

This bottom-line Best Question cuts to the core of assessing how patient centered this doctor is. The doctors who are strongly patient centered are more likely to explain treatment options and possible side effects. The best doctors will gladly answer all your questions at any time without exasperation or impatience and will encourage you to learn more about heart disease, risks, and prevention.

A doctor who enjoys giving you full and educational explanations is the most likely to treat you with respect. The best doctors encourage questions. In turn, the most knowledgeable patients are usually the most satisfied with their doctor and their care.

6. Did this doctor openly respect your opinions and decisions? Did you ever feel the doctor was talking down to you?

This question helps you to further assess this doctor's attitude and how opinionated he might be when presenting care options. Some people prefer a directive doctor who tells them what to do, whereas others prefer to do their own research and make independent decisions with the doctor's input.

There's no right or wrong way here. Just look for a doctor who is a good match for your own communication style.

7. How well did this doctor support you and your healing process after surgery and over time?

You don't want a surgeon who just cuts and runs. Likewise, your cardiologist should be your genuine ally. Asking this question of someone who is already a heart patient or heart attack survivor will go a long way in helping you to set your expectations for quality care and open communication with this particular doctor.

Press gently for more details including how well the doctor handled unexpected complications or advised about lifestyle changes or new treatments. Look for a partner, not just a doctor.

Kathy Berra, MNS, a clinical director at Stanford University's Heart Network, says, "Doctors who have nurse practitioners, physician assistants, and other professionals like dietitians working for them are the physicians who really recognize that it does take a village to take care of heart disease."

8. When your partner, family members, or friends accompanied you on office visits, did this doctor also include them in the discussion?

This is another question to determine how compassionate and patient centered this doctor is. If he values his patients from a whole-person perspective, it makes sense that the patient's family will be more readily folded into the discussions and decision making.

Good signs are a doctor who looks at everyone in the room when explaining something, asks others if they have questions, and encourages taking notes or making tape recordings of the meeting.

9. How accessible was this doctor or office staff after hours or on short notice?

Some doctors are generous with their after-hours time, offering you their cell phone number or personal e-mail address so that you can reach them anytime. Ask the person giving the referral to share any related stories so that you can be realistic about how accessible this doctor will be.

10. How well did this doctor's office staff treat you? Did you ever feel frustrated because of office inefficiency or long wait times to see the doctor?

There's a wide variation in office staff and their responsiveness to patients' needs. You are probably feeling pretty fragile right now, and the last thing you need in your life is a haughty, hostile receptionist or nurse in your doctor's office. You know the one. She acts like it will take an act of divine intervention before she finally agrees to copy a one-page report for your personal files.

You will be depending on this office staff to make sure office appointments are timely, your medical insurance carrier has been properly billed, and your medical records get into all the right hands.

❯ The Magic Question

Do you trust this doctor enough to send your own family to her? Why or why not?

This question works well whether you are asking a doctor or a friend for a referral. Trust is an intangible quality and not something that is easily earned.

Just be aware that the response to this "trust test" question is purely subjective. If you don't fully trust the person you are getting the referral from (think Ms. Yellow Pages), be sure to ask the follow-up question, "Why or why not?"

CONCLUSION

By the time you've asked these Best Questions, you'll have come a long way, baby, from just getting the prospective doctor's name and

IN SEARCH OF A DOCTOR I CAN TRUST

It's very important that you have a doctor you trust to help you manage your heart disease effectively. This is a lifelong condition. If you dislike your doctor, you are less likely to follow his advice and keep going to regular checkups.

Dr. Kim Allan Williams, a senior Chicago-based cardiologist and the current chairperson of the board for the Association of Black Cardiologists, comments, "There's a fair amount of fear for some African-Americans in their relationships with their physicians that often is not expressed."

Dr. Rebecca Allison, a Phoenix cardiologist and the 2009 president of the Gay and Lesbian Medical Association, says, "The main concern for a lot of gay, lesbian, bisexual, and transgender patients is being able to confide in their doctors. Many of us are fearful that our doctors will not be very receptive to us."

If these concerns sound familiar or you want a different doctor for other reasons, use the Best Questions in chapters 3 and 4 as your guide. Your heart deserves the best.

number. These Best Questions are like the key to unlocking your referral person's personal experiences with a doctor in a way that will be helpful to you without burdening her.

Now you are ready to make your first appointment with a new cardiologist or cardiac surgeon. Don't be tempted to rush past this important preliminary step in your quest for great doctoring. You deserve it. Chapter 4 provides your script for that first visit.

THE 10 BEST RESOURCES

American Heart Association. "Doctors, What to Consider When Choosing." www.americanheart.org/presenter.jhtml?identifier=4541.

American Medical Association. "Making the Most of an Office Visit." In *American Medical Association Guide to Talking to Your Doctor.* New York: John Wiley and Sons, 2001.

Centers for Medicare and Medicaid. "Choosing a Doctor: A Guide for People with Medicare." http://jobfunctions.bnet.com/whitepaper.aspx?docid =121268. (Registration required.)

Consumers' Checkbook. "Medical Advice: Is Your Doctor Measuring Up?" www.checkbook.org. (Subscription required.)

Groopman, Jerome. *How Doctors Think.* Boston: Houghton Mifflin, 2007.

HealthGrades. "Research Physicians." www.healthgrades.com. (Charges small fee.)

Manning, Phil R., and Lois DeBakey. *Medicine: Preserving the Passion in the 21st Century,* 2nd ed. Warren, MI: Springer, 2003.

National Institute on Aging. "Talking with Your Doctor: A Guide for Older People." www.nia.nih.gov/HealthInformation/Publications/Talking WithYourDoctor/.

Roizen, Michael F., and Mehmet C. Oz. *YOU: The Smart Patient: An Insider's Handbook for Getting the Best Treatment.* New York: Free Press, 2006.

Roter, Debra L., and Judith A. Hall. *Doctors Talking with Patients/Patients Talking with Doctors: Improving Communication in Medical Visits.* Westport, CT: Auburn House, 1992.

CHAPTER 4: THE 10 BEST QUESTIONS

To Find a Top Cardiologist
or Cardiac Surgeon

The good physician treats the disease; the great physician treats the patient who has the disease.
—William Osler, Canadian physician

Most of us believe that our lives might one day depend on the right decision by a doctor, a belief we have about few other professions. As you face the suddenness of a heart attack or the seriousness of a diagnosis of heart disease, that "one day" is no longer abstract. You need Dr. Right—right now.

But before you can proceed, you need to know how to find a really good cardiologist or cardiac surgeon. Having a top doctor can make a world of difference in your treatment and care options, lifestyle changes, and quality of life from now on.

But how do you find a great doctor? Finding a top cardiologist and/or heart surgeon may seem like a scary and daunting task unless you happen to have a brother-in-law who is one.

When describing their worst experiences with doctors, patients often cite arrogance, dismissive attitudes, and callousness rather than lack of technical expertise, Ohio State University researchers found in a 2006 study at the Mayo Clinic. So not only do you need a technically capable doctor, but also one with whom you can feel comfortable and who will treat you and your need for knowledge about heart disease with respect and dignity.

In his book, *How Doctors Think,* Dr. Jerome Groopman says that the attributes of the best doctors are a relish for knowledge, an insatiable curiosity, pride in their performance, and a "clear, clean joy in sharing with you their knowledge." He cites among the worst

---

THE QUESTION DOCTOR SAYS:

Be sure to tell your doctor at the beginning of your appointment that you have a list of questions and ask when she prefers to answer them. This way you'll know her preference for timing and will have politely informed her that you want enough time to get your questions answered.

---

attributes a doctor's unwillingness to listen, cynicism, and the tendency to treat all patients the same with "cookie-cutter" or one-size-fits-all treatments.

Even if you prefer to stay with a family doctor for ongoing cardiac care, you owe it to yourself to seek a second opinion (which is often covered by insurance carriers) from a cardiologist about your heart disease so that you can avoid future regrets or doubts. The 10 Best Questions in this chapter will help you choose the right person. Remember that the best doctors will welcome your questions and your desire to choose a doctor or surgeon carefully. If a doctor reacts negatively to your questions or refuses to answer them, consider this a red flag. This doctor either has something to hide or may be impatient with you during future office visits.

>>> THE 10 BEST QUESTIONS
To Find a Top Cardiologist or Cardiac Surgeon

1. Are you board-certified? What are your other medical credentials?

Board certification matters. Board certification assures you that the doctor has passed the board requirements for her specialty. In the United States, medical specialty certification is voluntary. Doctors receive their medical licenses after completing medical school and residency requirements. But this doesn't apply to medical specialties like cardiology, and only sets the minimum competency requirements to treat patients.

THE QUESTION DOCTOR SAYS:

If you feel shy or intimidated about asking a potential doctor about credentials, ask the office staff, go to the doctor's Web site or bio, or simply do your own search using the resources in this chapter. If you are satisfied about a doctor's credentials, skip asking this question in person.

But don't skip question 1 altogether just because it seems hard to ask. You don't want someone who has served jail time for malpractice operating on you or prescribing medications!

The successful completion of the examinations for board certification demonstrates a doctor's exceptional expertise and his or her dedication to a rigorous, voluntary commitment to lifelong learning. This is especially important with heart disease, because of the need to stay current with fast-moving research advances in this field. To maintain board certification, doctors must complete specialty training and periodic exams to demonstrate their ongoing competency. Use the search services of the American Board of Medical Specialties (www.abms.org) to check for a specific doctor's certification.

A valid state license is also very important. Go to the American Medical Association's Web site for links to your state's medical board (www.ama-assn.org/ama/pub/category/2645.html).

Checking on past disciplinary actions and malpractice suits is tougher because most medical professionals don't readily disclose unclean histories. See ChoiceTrust (www.choicetrust.com) or HealthGrades (www.healthgrades.com), two comprehensive Web sites that charge a small fee for their services. Other sources for checking on prior complaints or disciplinary actions are free at Administrators in Medicine (http://docboard.org) and Health Care Choices (www.healthcarechoices.org).

SKILLFUL HEART SURGEONS

Asking a heart surgeon how many times he has performed surgery is absolutely vital. Smart surgical skills honed from doing hundreds or even thousands of surgeries or procedures are your best insurance for a successful surgery and recovery. Remember, the more experience, the better. You want a surgeon who is so experienced that your surgery is just another routine day in the operating room for him.

Stanford University Heart Network's clinical director Kathy Berra shares her deep wisdom from thirty-five years of cardiac care. "What makes a really great surgeon is his outcomes — his death rate. Most hospitals report their death rates from heart surgery and other surgeries. These rates can be compared to the national average. Obviously, you will want to go to a hospital [and surgeon] with a very low death rate."

2. What is your experience with my type of heart disease? How many patients like me did you see during the past twelve months?

Experience matters, too—a lot. The number of years of total medical practice is significant, along with the years of specialized practice a doctor has in treating heart disease.

It's very important to determine a doctor's or a surgeon's prior experience with heart disease, cardiac interventions, or surgeries. One way to determine a doctor's specialized expertise is to ask, "How many surgeries do you do a month?" or "What percentage of your practice is devoted to treating heart patients?" The higher the number, the better it is for you.

If you live in a rural community or have limited access to specialized care centers, doctors will naturally have lower yearly numbers. In this case, ask this question as a percentage of this doctor's total practice.

A good bedside manner can be very comforting. But don't choose a doctor based on personality alone. A doctor's personality should be your secondary—not primary—consideration in making your choice.

3. May I speak to at least one of your patients to see how he or she made out in these same circumstances?

This Best Question was suggested by former surgeon general Dr. C. Everett Koop. He believes it's very important to follow through on patient referrals.

Asking for a referral is more common than you might think. Be sure to follow through and make the phone calls. Chapter 3 gives you specific Best Questions for getting highly reliable referrals.

4. Which hospitals are you affiliated with?

You have two choices: You can choose your doctor first and then go with the hospital where she has admitting privileges. Or you can choose the hospital or heart disease center first and then find a top doctor there.

In the second scenario, you will be focused on the facility's expertise or reputation over an individual doctor's skills. Either way, ask this follow-up question: "What is the accreditation status of this hospital or medical facility?" See chapter 11 on hospitals. Note that if you live in a rural area or choose not to travel for treatments, your choices may be more limited.

5. Are you affiliated with any medical schools?

A teaching affiliation with a prestigious medical school is the gold standard when looking for a top cardiologist. It's a fairly reliable indicator that a doctor is considered by her peers to be a leader in this field.

Academic doctors who also practice medicine are likely to be the most well informed about the latest in heart-disease research, diagnostic tools, and treatments, and they will keep current through frequent contacts with their medical colleagues.

6. Are you involved with any ongoing research projects or clinical trials on heart disease?

Experts suggest that you look for doctors who have written about heart disease cases similar to yours and whose work is often cited in medical journals. If a doctor you are considering has been published, ask for copies of those articles. Even if the articles are written for medical professionals and are very technical, you can learn a lot about this doctor's interests and approach to treating heart disease. Go to PubMed Central (www.pubmedcentral.nih.gov) for a free archive of medical journal abstracts.

7. What percentage of your patients who are heart attack survivors like me do you refer to a cardiac rehabilitation program?

Your doctor's answer to this question will reveal two things: (1) You'll know more about how committed this doctor is to supporting your long-term recovery through the lifestyle changes you'll need for lifelong good heart health. (2) You want to hear from this doctor that she refers at least 50 percent of her patients to cardiac rehabilitation.

The national average for cardiac rehab referrals is about 50 percent, and you'll be smart to be part of that statistic. Younger men get more referrals than older women, so be sure to add the phrase "like me" to your question. See chapter 12 on the importance of cardiac rehabilitation.

8. How will you keep my family involved in care decisions? Do you offer support services and more information about heart disease?

The doctor's answer to this question will indicate if she is patient centered and family centered. You want a doctor who considers you and your family as unique individuals.

Dr. Timothy J. Gardner, president of the American Heart Association, says, "The patient and his family need to understand that even in the throes of a medical crisis they can still expect the physician to be patient with them and give them the chance to examine all medical options." George Washington University's Dr. Christina M. Puchalski adds, "The mark of a good doctor is someone who can treat every patient as an individual and not make hasty conclusions from preconceived notions."

If you have choices, go to a doctor who emphasizes cardiac rehabilitation and offers referrals to support services, such as specially trained cardiac nurses, physical therapists, nutritionists, and family counselors. The best doctors are also good teachers. As former acting U.S. surgeon general rear admiral Dr. Kenneth P. Moritsugu comments, "When the doctor seeks to educate the patient, they are not merely engaging in a two-way conversation. Rather, the doctor is taking it beyond the conversation in order to teach the patient about their medical options and how to take control of his or her own health and well-being."

9. Please describe your preferences for communicating with your patients.

Communication obstacles rank high on patients' list of complaints. Most people highly value how well a doctor communicates with both the patient and his family, especially if your primary caregiver is directly and personally involved with your recovery after your heart attack.

10. Who covers for you when you aren't available or are on vacation?

This is another question that most patients don't think to ask until they can't reach their doctor when they really need to.

Be sure that your doctor tells you how she will communicate

with you if unanticipated problems come up or when she's unavailable or on vacation. Also ask how (calls or e-mails) and when (best times of day) she can be reached.

❯ The Magic Question

What is the last thing you learned about heart disease?

The best answer to this question is not so much what the doctor says but how easily the response rolls off her tongue.

If this doctor is truly an excellent doctor and sees plenty of heart patients, she'll be able to easily say something like, "Well, I read an article last week" or "I went to a conference last month." But if she is groping for an answer, look elsewhere for your cardiologist or surgeon. You don't want your doctor to be the last one to know about new heart disease research discoveries and improved therapies.

CONCLUSION

If a prospective doctor obviously enjoys—passionately enjoys—the practice of medicine, shows evidence of following new developments, thinks hard about you and your problems, asks questions of you, shows a real interest in your answers, and meets the requirements for board certification and experience, you probably have a very good doctor or surgeon. From the group of good doctors that you find, choose a doctor you can trust and feel comfortable with.

Dr. Kenneth P. Moritsugu concludes, "A lot of people say, 'Talk to your doctor about this or that.' I think the preposition *to* is wrong. It's talking *with* your health professional. It's subtle but sends a very, very clear message that *talking with* is an adult-to-adult relationship, an equal partnership."

THE 10 BEST RESOURCES

American Board of Medical Specialties. "Is Your Doctor Certified?" Board certification for doctors. www.abms.org/wc/login.aspx.

American Heart Association. "Surgery and Other Medical Procedures: How to Find a Surgeon." www.americanheart.org/presenter.jhtml?identifier=123.

American Medical Association. "Doctor Finder." www.ama-assn.org/aps/amahg.htm. (Search this major database by the state where a doctor practices medicine.)

Consumers' Checkbook. "Guide to Top Doctors." www.checkbook.org. (Subscription required.)

Consumers Union of U.S. "Doctor, Can We Talk? (How to Develop a Good Relationship with a New Physician)." *Special Report for Consumer Reports on Health.* July 2001.

Groopman, Jerome. "Epilogue: A Patient's Questions." In *How Doctors Think.* Boston: Houghton Mifflin, 2007.

HealthGrades. "Find a Physician." www.healthgrades.com. (Charges small fee.)

Leeds, Dorothy. *Smart Questions to Ask Your Doctor.* New York: Harper Paperbacks, 1992.

Manning, Phil R., and Lois DeBakey "Reading: Keeping Current." In *Medicine: Preserving the Passion in the 21st Century,* 2nd ed. New York: Springer, 2003.

Rimmerman, Curtis M. *You and Your Cardiologist: A Cleveland Clinic Guide.* Cleveland: Cleveland Clinic Press, 2008.

CHAPTER 5: THE 10 BEST QUESTIONS

For Understanding Diagnostic Tests and Cardiac Procedures

He who has health, has hope; and he who has hope, has everything.

—Norwegian proverb

If you've already had a heart attack or a very close call, chances are you've already had numerous diagnostic tests and procedures on your heart's current condition and prognosis. The typical tests used to diagnose a heart attack include an electrocardiogram (ECG), cardiac blood tests, echocardiography, cardiac catheterization, and angiography. Each test is explained in this chapter. See also chapter 1.

Perhaps you've been admitted to the hospital with severe angina (chest pains). Or maybe you've been told you have coronary artery disease or are at high risk for a heart attack. If so, you want to take all the precautions possible including getting all the right tests and procedures.

As cardiologist and medical director Dr. Mimi Guarneri at the Scripps Center for Integrative Medicine in La Jolla, California, says, "You need to educate yourself. You can use your physician for guidance, but you need to educate yourself, too." Dr. Alfred Bove, president of the American College of Cardiology and a professor emeritus at the Temple University Medical Center, adds his advice: "There are national guidelines for tests that should be provided to all patients after a heart attack."

The two broad categories of diagnostic tests and procedures for heart disease are **noninvasive** and **invasive**. A noninvasive test means that there are no instruments or fluids inserted in your body,

---

THE QUESTION DOCTOR SAYS:

Don't be afraid to learn more about your heart disease and diagnostic tests. It's what you don't know that can hurt you. You aren't expected by anyone — your doctors, your partner, your loved ones, or yourself — to be a genius about heart disease. All you need are the right questions. Let your doctor come up with the right answers.

---

whereas an invasive test is the opposite. Some procedures, like coronary angioplasties, are nonsurgical invasive tests and are also commonly used to treat blocked arteries.

Usually doctors will start with simple tests. But their choice of tests depends on your medical history, risk factors, current symptoms, and assessed problems. You may have some input, but most people rely on their doctors' expertise and guidance, especially during a heart attack or other emergency situation.

Regardless of your heart's current status, the following Best Questions will prepare you for talking over your options with your doctor and making sure she hasn't forgotten to tell you something. There's also a quick guide and explanation of the major diagnostic tests and procedures.

>>>THE 10 BEST QUESTIONS
For Understanding Diagnostic Tests and Cardiac Procedures

1. Why do I need this test or procedure?
Get specifics including why this test or procedure is personally good for you and not just that it's routinely done for most heart patients.

2. Are there any alternatives or less invasive procedures that are equally effective?

Ideally, you want your doctor to perform noninvasive tests as a first choice.

3. How many times have you done this test or procedure?

Asking this important question ensures that your doctor or medical technician is experienced enough to handle any unforeseen problems or emergencies.

4. How is it done?

Expect to get a detailed description, including whether you'll be sedated, how you will be prepped for the procedure, how long it will take, and what you need to do in advance to prepare, including continuing or stopping your medications, food, and drink.

5. Will it hurt during the test/procedure or afterward?

If you want more than a yes/no answer, ask the doctor how the average patient would rate this test/procedure on the standard pain scale (1 is no pain; 10 is excruciating pain).

6. Are there any side effects?

Side effects vary widely with the complexity of the test, whether it's an invasive procedure, and your physical condition.

7. What happens afterward?

Ask your doctor to explain in detail your recovery, including if you can drive home yourself. Also ask, "Will I have to have this test repeated again later?" and "What if I experience the same chest discomfort or symptoms after the procedure?"

8. How soon will I get the results?

This answer will depend on the type of test or procedure and how the results are analyzed.

9. When and how will you explain the results and your recommendations?

Ask if you'll need to make a separate office appointment to discuss the results. Expect your doctor to give you a well-balanced explanation with several options for treatment. Ask specifically, "Do I have coronary artery disease?" If so, ask, "How many blockages do I have?" and "Where are the blockages located?"

10. Where can I get more information about my heart disease or this procedure?

Some cardiologists provide brochures or have staff willing to answer your questions. Also check with the American Heart Association (www.americanheart.org or call 1-800-242-8721).

> The Magic Question

Are there any possible complications from this test that won't go away quickly or at all?

This question may not apply to a simple noninvasive test. But if you are having an invasive procedure, this long-shot question is in the category of better safe than sorry.

If you are a high-risk patient, are older, or have already had a heart attack, ask, "Is there any chance this procedure might cause a heart attack?"

Another Magic Question is suggested by Dr. Spencer King, III, an executive director and the interim president of the Saint Joseph's Heart and Vascular Institute in Atlanta. His advice is, if it is not an emergency situation that you ask, "Is this a test to find out what I have or is this a test and treatment? If the doctor says, 'Well, if I find something there, I'll just fix it,' I don't like that answer very much. I'd get a second opinion."

Due to the complexity of heart tests and their objectives, it can be very confusing for patients to fully understand the overall purpose of a recommended test, such as cardiac catheterization, which is used for both treatment and diagnostic purposes. You also want to understand beforehand if you have the option of taking medication instead of having an invasive procedure.

SUMMARY OF DIAGNOSTIC TESTS

Noninvasive Tests and Procedures

Electrocardiogram

The electrocardiogram (ECG or EKG) is a simple, common, quick, and painless test that traces your heart's electrical activity. A more detailed type of ECG is the **signal-averaged electrocardiogram (SAECG)**.

Ambulatory electrocardiogram

An ambulatory electrocardiogram records your heart's electrical activity while you do your usual activities. Many people's irregular heartbeats (arrhythmias) are noticeable only during certain times, like exercise, eating, or even sleeping. Also called **Holter monitoring** and **cardiac event monitoring**.

Stress/exercise electrocardiogram

The patient rides a stationary bike or walks on a treadmill to determine if there is a blocked artery, to evaluate chest pains or arrhythmias, and to measure the heart's strength and post–heart attack functioning.

Echocardiogram

An echocardiogram uses painless sound waves to see if your heart is enlarged, weakened, or has a damaged valve.

Vascular ultrasound

This is a general term for ultrasound tests to see your veins and arteries, monitor blood flow, identify blockages, and evaluate your suitability for an angioplasty or a coronary artery bypass graft. A special type is the **Doppler ultrasound** to evaluate blood flow. Another type, **lower extremity arterial ultrasound,** is used for patients with peripheral arterial disease (PAD). **Noninvasive flow studies** also look for PAD for people who have pain while walking. **Carotid ultrasound** looks for atherosclerosis in the neck arteries and a blockage condition called **carotid stenosis.**

Computerized tomography (CT) scan

CT scans can detect coronary artery disease and congenital heart disease and help to evaluate your heart prior to a more complex procedure.

Electron beam computed tomography (EBCT)

EBCT x-rays evaluate bypass grafts, cardiac lesions, and cardiac functioning. EBCT also measures calcium deposits in the coronary arteries.

Cardiac positron emission tomography (PET)

PET scans can accurately detect coronary artery disease, heart muscle injuries, and other heart functions.

CT angiography

Also called **digital cardiac angiography (DCA)** or **digital subtraction angiography (DSA),** this imaging test uses injected dye to show if there are blockages and their severity.

Cardiac magnetic resonance imaging (MRI)

MRIs evaluate your heart's structure and functions. They can detect coronary artery disease, heart failure, congenital heart disease, and rare heart conditions. A special type of MRI is called **magnetic resonance angiography (MRA)** and is less invasive than traditional angioplasties.

Single-photon emission computed tomography (SPECT)

A SPECT test is a nuclear medicine technique that uses a gamma camera to provide three-dimensional images of the heart's functions, thickness, and other diagnostic information.

Enhanced external counterpulsation (EECP)

This procedure helps to restore blood flow to the heart, relieves chest pain (angina) and ischemia, and lowers the risk of a heart attack or other heart problems.

Invasive Tests and Procedures

Blood tests

There are numerous blood tests to confirm that a heart attack has occurred, determine the extent of heart damage and coronary artery disease (CAD), predict your future risk for heart problems, and choose your best treatment plan. These blood tests measure cardiac enzymes (such as troponin and creatine kinase), C-reactive protein, fibrinogen, homocysteine, lipoproteins, triglycerides, brain natriuretic peptide, and prothrombin.

Cardiac catheterization

This term describes a general group of nonsurgical procedures done in a cardiac catheterization laboratory by a specialized team of cardiologists and technicians. These diagnostic procedures are widely used for detecting and treating narrowed or blocked arteries, measuring blood pressure within the heart and oxygen in the blood, and evaluating heart muscle function.

Coronary angiogram

Also known as angiography or arteriography, this special x-ray helps to detect if your coronary arteries are blocked, where, and by how much. This is one of the most common and definitive cardiac diagnostic tests. It is done by inserting a thin tube (catheter) into an artery and up to the heart.

Transesophageal echocardiography

During this ultrasound test a tube is passed through the throat and into the esophagus in order to evaluate the heart's functioning and gather information about abnormal heart rhythms (arrhythmias).

Electrophysiologic test

Catheters are used to locate and analyze arrhythmias in different parts of the heart.

Thallium stress test

This type of exercise stress test uses an injected radioactive substance (thallium) to help determine heart attack damage, coronary artery blockage, arrhythmias, and the causes of chest pain (angina). It is also known as myocardial perfusion imaging (MPI), multigated acquisition (MUGA) scan, radionuclide stress test, and nuclear stress test.

CONCLUSION

There is no single, simple test for heart disease. Understanding the tests and procedures recommended by your doctor is critical. They hold the key to your diagnosis, treatment plan, and prognosis.

Let your doctor educate you by giving you his best answers to your Best Questions. Don't be afraid to ask questions, including your own. You deserve a full explanation in simple language about what the proposed test involves, why it's important, possible side effects, and recovery.

THE 10 BEST RESOURCES

American Heart Association. "Diagnosing Heart Disease." www.americanheart.org/presenter.jhtml?identifier=330.

American Heart Association. "Tests to Diagnose Heart Disease." www.americanheart.org/presenter.jhtml?identifier=4739.

American Heart Association. "Treatment Options." www.americanheart .org/presenter.jhtml?identifier=1598.

American Heart Association. "Treatments and Tests." www.american heart.org/presenter.jhtml?identifier=3004353.

Australian Government. National Health and Medical Research Council. "Making Decisions About Tests and Treatments." www.nhmrc.gov.au/ publications/synopses/_files/hpr25.pdf.

British Heart Foundation. "Tests for your Heart." www.bhf.org.uk/publi cations.aspx.

Cleveland Clinic Foundation. "Tests and Procedures." http://my.cleve landclinic.org/heart/services/tests/default.aspx.

Consumer Health Reports. "Too Much Treatment?" June 2008. www .consumers.org. (Subscription required.)

Margolis, Simeon. *The Johns Hopkins Consumer Guide to Medical Tests: What You Can Expect, How You Should Prepare, What Your Results Mean.* New York: Medletter Associates, 2001.

WebMD. "Heart Disease Guide: Diagnosis and Tests." www.webmd.com/ heart-disease/guide/heart-disease-diagnosis-tests.

CHAPTER 6: THE 10 BEST QUESTIONS
To Ask When Getting a Second Opinion

No doctor is better than two or three.

—German proverb

Seriously consider getting a second opinion if your diagnosis is for a chronic disease (judged incurable), a life-threatening condition, a rare disorder, or because you don't like or trust your current doctor. You may also want a second opinion about your laboratory report, prescription medications, treatment plan, or almost any aspect of your medical care.

There are twin trends for more second opinion requests. Patients are getting more involved, empowered, and knowledgeable about their own medical care. With the exploding field of medical science, there are also more treatment options than ever before for just about every disease known to humankind.

The good news is that most insurance plans and Medicare will pay for second and even third opinions for life-threatening conditions such as heart disease. For some cases, insurance plans even require second opinions. Check with your health care provider on specific policies for your condition.

Even though it may take additional time and effort to locate and see another doctor, a delay for this purpose usually won't impact your prognosis. Make sure you verify this with your doctor when you are discussing your medical condition and the timing of your treatment plan.

If you are seeing a primary care physician who has limited experience with your medical condition, consider getting a second opinion from a top specialist or medical center experienced in treating this disease. See chapters 3 and 4 for finding and choosing a medical specialist.

Don't worry about offending your current doctor or challenging his expertise. The best doctors welcome second opinions and even seek out additional advice. If your current doctor strongly objects, his reaction may be a red flag that he lacks experience or self-confidence in treating your disease. Dr. Spencer B. King, III, an executive director and the interim president of the Saint Joseph's Heart and Vascular Institute in Atlanta, says, "Second opinions are the same as getting a couple of estimates for redoing your kitchen. The cost might be the same, but different people have different ideas on what needs to be done."

Remember, it's your health and well-being that's ultimately at stake here. Dr. Vicki Rackner, a patient advocate and a co-author of the book *Heart Disease* in the *Chicken Soup for the Soul: Healthy Living* series, is a strong believer in the value of second opinions. She says simply, "You need a second opinion for everything."

This chapter's Best Questions are a little different. Ask *yourself* the first five Best Questions to help you decide if you really want a second opinion, especially if you must pay for it yourself. Ask the *second-opinion doctor* questions 6 through 10 when you are meeting with her to discuss your case.

>>> THE 5 BEST QUESTIONS
To Ask Yourself *Before Seeking a Second Opinion*

1. How do I rate my current doctor's knowledge about my disease and her ability to support me well during treatment?

Many patients underestimate what they should know about their disease and its treatment. At your initial diagnosis, you probably didn't know much about your disease and its complexities.

Medical specialists, such as cardiologists, neurologists, dermatologists, and psychiatrists, will be more knowledgeable in their specialties than your primary care physician. You want a doctor you can count on, especially if your disease is chronic (incurable), life-threatening, or impacts your quality of life.

2. How confident am I in my current doctor's interest in treating me as a unique person?

You're trying to assess if your current doctor is a great, good, or just a mediocre doctor. Think back to your doctor's treatment plan for you. How comprehensive was it? Did she seem sincerely interested in you as an individual? Did she fully explain your treatment options? Do you feel you can trust her?

By all means, avoid highly opinionated doctors who prescribe the same drugs or surgical procedure over and over again for most of their patients. Legendary psychologist Abraham Maslow once noted that when all you have is a hammer, everything looks like a nail. The same applies here. When a doctor only knows a small handful of treatment options, every patient looks the same—like a nail with heart disease.

3. How much do I understand about what I've been told to date about my diagnosis and treatment options?

Reflect on your prior discussions with your doctor. Look over your notes. Scan this book to learn more about treatment options. All of this will help the factual information to sink in as you step back to assess your situation for a moment.

Now with this clear head, think through how much you truly understand. This is not a reflection on your intelligence but rather a sign of how well your current doctor has explained your diagnosis and treatment plan.

You want a doctor who is willing and capable of putting medical jargon into easy-to-understand terms. The word *doctor* is from the Latin *docere,* meaning "to teach." The medical profession has evolved over time, and now we think of doctoring and teaching as two separate functions. But look for a good doctor who is also willing to be your teacher.

4. How complicated is my diagnosis and treatment plan?

If you think you have a straightforward medical case, don't assume you don't need to make any decisions or educate yourself. In most cases you still have choices, such as where you want to be treated. For example, 75 percent of elderly men in one Maine town had prostate surgery compared to only 25 percent of similar cases in a nearby town, according to studies done by Dartmouth Medical School.

The beliefs, customs, financial practices, medical education, and available resources are behind-the-scenes factors that influence a doctor's decisions and are usually not obvious to patients. Your doctor's recommendations are based on his subjective assessment of your case. Doctors are only human and can make mistakes.

5. What does my inner voice tell me is right for me?

There's a lot to be said for the value of going with your gut-level reaction. After you've asked all the highly logical, rational, analytical questions, you should also listen to your inner voice.

Malcolm Gladwell, the author of *Blink,* would agree. He says, "We really only trust conscious decision making. But there are moments, particularly in times of stress, when haste does not make waste, when our snap judgments and first impressions can offer a much better means of making sense of the world. . . . Decisions made very quickly can be every bit as good as decisions made cautiously and deliberately."

THE QUESTION DOCTOR SAYS

Use questions 6 through 10 to ask a second-opinion doctor about your diagnosis and treatments, or just to find a doctor you'll like better. Before you begin your doctor search, get a clear idea of what kind of doctor you want and why.

⟩⟩⟩THE 5 BEST QUESTIONS
To Ask the Doctor *When Getting a Second Opinion*

6. How do you interpret my test results?

Ask the second doctor to review the test results to give you his interpretation of the diagnosis. Medical experts and patients disagree about whether your second opinion should be "blind." A blind second opinion means that the first doctor's opinion and sometimes the original test results aren't shared with the second doctor.

The advantage is that the blind second opinion will be more objective and not influenced by the first one. The drawbacks include putting your second-opinion doctor at a disadvantage by not letting him know the basis for the original diagnosis. Another option is to provide test results and other information without including the first doctor's diagnosis and treatment recommendations.

7. What are the chances that my test results could indicate a different diagnosis?

If your initial heart disease diagnosis is complex or not definitive, it may be at least partially wrong. In a 1997 survey commissioned by the National Patient Safety Foundation, 42 percent of those surveyed reported a past medical mistake, misdiagnosis, or treatment error. Misdiagnosis rates in a hospital's ICU or emergency department are estimated to be between 20 and 40 percent.

8. In your opinion, has my disease been properly diagnosed and described? Please explain the rationale for your answer.

This is a straightforward question that goes to the heart of why you want a second opinion. Make sure the second doctor takes the time to fully explain her reasoning behind her assessment of your situation. Don't hesitate to ask any other questions in order to understand what you're being told.

9. Are there any alternative forms of treatment available that my previous doctor may have overlooked? What treatments do you recommend for me?

Not all doctors are equally supportive of alternative therapies, such as healthy diet and exercise choices, acupuncture, aromatherapy, and dietary supplements. But there is growing evidence-based research within the context of rigorous science that some complementary and alternative treatments have value (also called **integrative medicine**).

The federal government's National Center for Complementary and Alternative Medicine has an informative Web site (http://nccam.nih.gov). See also chapter 13. A second opinion that includes a look at alternative or complementary treatments may expand your healing options in ways that a primary care physician or medical specialist hadn't previously considered.

10. In your opinion, what is my prognosis after going through the treatment plan you've outlined? What is my risk of a recurrence of this disease?

Try to refrain from asking this question too early in the discussion. This way you can really listen to everything else the doctor has to

THE QUESTION DOCTOR SAYS:

Reduce the cost and time required for a second opinion by asking your first doctor to send copies of all test results to the second-opinion doctor if you choose not to have a blind second opinion. Take a friend or family member, a notepad, and a tape recorder to this office visit. That way you'll be able to listen and can compare notes and recordings later between the first and second doctors.

say and make a well-informed decision about whether you like his treatment plan, personal style, and potential to support you in the upcoming months. Pay attention to how detailed and personalized his answer is to this question.

> The Magic Question

What advice would you give to your mother (sister, wife) to help her choose between the different recommendations/diagnoses/treatment options I've received?

If the first and second doctors disagree on the diagnosis or treatment plan, you may be confronted with a situation in which you have to choose between them without really knowing which one is better.

Rather than trying to be the Lone Ranger here and solve this problem yourself, this Magic Question will put the second-opinion doctor's thinking cap on and engage him in helping you make the best decision. If needed, you can also go back to your first doctor and ask this same question and then compare answers.

Another strategy is to ask the two doctors to confer on your case and see if they can arrive at a mutual decision. You might also want to ask for a third opinion and then compare.

CONCLUSION

Why get a second opinion? The fundamental question when you are considering second opinions is really, "Why not?" As Mayo Clinic's cardiologist Dr. Sharonne Hayes says, "I tell a lot of women that they should get a second opinion regardless, especially if there's anything unusual about their medical history. Most doctors welcome second opinions."

Asking for a second opinion is a frequent practice, growing more common, and some insurance companies even recommend it. Don't worry about insulting a doctor's intelligence, even if he's your old favorite family doctor. The best doctors will actively support you. Oftentimes, patients choose to stay with their first doctor after seeking a second opinion.

A heart attack is a frightening event and treating heart disease can be complex. You deserve to have all the information and support you need to help you deal with it. Seeking a second opinion may give you peace of mind, knowing that you've done everything possible to ensure an accurate diagnosis and the best care available.

THE 10 BEST RESOURCES

About.com. "Second Opinions: Why It's Important to Get a Second Opinion." http://lungdiseases.about.com/od/lungcancer/a/secondopinions.htm.

American Heart Association. "Second Medical Opinions." www.americanheart.org/presenter.jhtml?identifier=4703.

Centers for Medicare and Medicaid Services. "Getting a Second Opinion Before Surgery." www.medicare.gov/Publications/Pubs/pdf/02173.pdf.

Eldercare Team. "Getting a Second Opinion." www.eldercareteam.com/resources/articles/secondopinion.htm.

Gladwell, Malcolm. *Blink: The Power of Thinking Without Thinking.* New York: Little, Brown, 2005.

Groopman, Jerome. "The Uncertainty of the Expert." In *How Doctors Think.* Boston: Houghton Mifflin, 2007.

Gruman, Jessie. *AfterShock: What to Do When the Doctor Gives You—Or Someone You Love—a Devastating Diagnosis.* New York: Walker & Company, 2007.

Levine, Evan. *What Your Doctor Won't (or Can't) Tell You: The Failures of American Medicine—and How to Avoid Becoming a Statistic.* New York: Berkley Trade, 2005.

U.S. Department of Health and Human Services. Agency for Healthcare Research and Quality. "Quick Tips—When Talking with Your Doctor." www.ahrq.gov/consumer/quicktips/doctalk.htm.

Wrongdiagnosis.com. "How Common Is Misdiagnosis?" www.wrong diagnosis.com/intro/common.htm.

CHAPTER 7: THE 10 BEST QUESTIONS

About Managing Your Risk Factors for Heart Disease

> The doctor of the future will give no medicine, but will educate his patients in the care of the human frame, in diet, and in the cause and prevention of disease.
>
> —Thomas Edison

I f you have been told you have heart disease or have already had a heart attack, your follow-up visits with either your cardiologist or your family doctor are very important. You need to recruit your doctor to be a supportive ally as you take on the hard homework of making heart-healthy lifestyle changes.

Use the following Best Questions as a guide to your conversation with your doctor and to make sure he has remembered to tell you key points during your ongoing office visits. You may also have other health issues for which you'll need to develop your own specific questions.

>>> THE 10 BEST QUESTIONS
About Managing Your Risk Factors for Heart Disease

1. What is my ideal weight? How can I achieve it? What is my BMI? What is my hip-to-waist measurement?

Americans' expanding waistlines are a well known fact. Obesity has doubled since the 1970s, and now at least 62 percent of adults in the United States are overweight or obese. Nearly 70 percent of all cases of cardiovascular disease are related to obesity. The official definition of obese is being 30 or more pounds overweight.

The more you weigh, the more likely you are to have a heart at-

THE QUESTION DOCTORS SAYS:

Consider focusing on just one or two of these risk factors during each of your visits with your doctor if you want to have a more in-depth discussion. You might make better use of your time together by just discussing your weight, family history, or smoking, for example.

tack earlier in life. To properly assess your weight-related heart risks, you need three numbers: (1) your weight in pounds; (2) your body mass index (BMI), which is a key measure of obesity; and (3) your hip-to-waist ratio.

Ask your doctor for a body mass index (BMI) test, a simple, quick, and painless measure of your body's fatness. An ideal BMI is 25 or less. Someone with a BMI over 30 is considered obese.

A 2008 Duke University study of more than one hundred thousand people who had had heart attacks looked specifically at BMI. A significant link was found between BMI, obesity, and heart attack risk.

The average age at which a first heart attack occurs is directly correlated to an increasing BMI. For thin people with a BMI of 18.5 or less, it is 74.6 years. For people with a BMI of 25 to 30, their heart attacks occur 3.5 years earlier at age 71.1. People with BMIs between 30 and 35 have first heart attacks at the average age of 67.8. Those with BMIs between 35 to 40 are on average 65.2 years old (more than 9 years younger than thin people). But the worst of all are obese people with BMIs over 40. They have first heart attacks at an average age of only 58.7 years old.

Ask your doctor to measure your waist-to-hip ratio, which is also related to your body shape. People who carry most of their excessive weight around their waist (so-called apple shape) are at higher risk for heart disease than people who are heavier below their waist (pear shape). A waist-to-hip ratio greater than 0.9 percent (usually a waist of 40 inches or more) for men and 0.85 percent (usually a waist of 35 inches or more) for women indicates greater risk of heart disease.

Your hip-to-waist measurement is an important number to know. New studies published in the *Journal of the American College of Cardiology* found that waist-to-hip ratio was a better predictor of cardiovascular risks than BMI. Judge your own weight, BMI, and hip-to-waist ratio using the Centers for Disease Control and Prevention's Web site at www.cdc.gov/nccdphp/dnpa/healthyweight/assessing/index.htm.

Losing weight isn't easy. Ask your doctor for specific advice, follow the guidelines you receive in your cardiac rehabilitation program, and see chapter 15 in this book for diet tips.

2. What foods should I eat? What type of diet do you recommend for me?

Currently, the most commonly recommended diet is the Mediterranean diet filled with fruits, vegetables, fiber, grains, and healthy fish and oils.

One smart question that you might not think to ask your doctor is, "How can I take my favorite foods and make them healthier?" For example, Dr. Kim Allan Williams, a noted Chicago cardiologist and the current chairperson of the board for the Association of Black Cardiologists, suggests, "Take soul food, reduce the salt, and replace the meat with a soy product, such as soy sausages, chicken, or burgers. Use olive oil instead of lard. If you replace the meat, sodium, and lard, you're doing pretty well."

3. What are my cholesterol numbers for HDL, LDL, and triglycerides? What do my cholesterol numbers indicate about my heart risks? How can I improve my cholesterol?

Knowing your HDL, LDL, and triglyceride levels is an important step in being a well-informed heart patient. These are the three main blood particles that make up your total **lipid count,** or the fatty substances in your blood collectively called **cholesterol.** The cutting-edge research indicates that you should *not* focus on your total cholesterol number but rather know all three: HDL, LDL, and triglyceride levels.

With **HDL (good) cholesterol,** higher levels are better. Heart risks happen with low HDL levels (less than 40 mg/dL for men, less than 50 mg/dL for women). Normal levels range from 40 to 60 mg/dL. Above 60 mg/dL is considered heart protective.

The lower your **LDL (bad) cholesterol,** the lower your risk of heart disease. LDL cholesterol is the bad fat in your arteries. Less than 100 mg/dL is optimal, and a level of 190 mg/dL and above is a very high risk. (Associate H with high and L with low to remember the difference between the "good" and "bad" cholesterols.)

Triglycerides are a type of fat. The normal level is less than 150 mg/dL, borderline high is 150–199 mg/dL, and too high is 200 mg/dL and up.

A toxic combination is low HDL (good) and high triglyceride levels. This is called **metabolic syndrome.** People with metabolic syndrome are at an extra high risk for developing heart disease and diabetes. See more at the American Heart Association's Web site: http://www.americanheart.org/presenter.jhtml?identifier=4756.

You can manage your cholesterol with a healthy diet, regular exercise, and sensible weight maintenance. All cholesterol abnormalities tend to improve with healthful lifestyle changes, especially reducing triglyceride levels.

Don't settle for just your total cholesterol number from your doctor. Ask her to explain the details of your profile. Blood cholesterol is complicated. For example, there are seven types of LDL (bad) cholesterol and five types of HDL (good) cholesterol.

In addition, many researchers now think that blood cholesterol is *not* the best predictor of heart disease risk. They believe there are other factors that cause heart attacks that may be more significant than cholesterol numbers. Some people who have heart attacks don't have high cholesterol levels.

Dr. H. Robert Superko, who led the major cholesterol study done in the 1980s at Stanford University and now heads research projects at St. Joseph's Translational Research Institute in Atlanta, explains, "Cholesterol is a major cause of heart disease in people who have high cholesterol, but most people don't have high cholesterol. What the drug companies want you to believe is that if you just take our drug (statins) you'll be fine. But the truth is that a 25 percent relative heart attack risk reduction is not good enough. This 25 percent reduction means that if one hundred people NOT taking the drug have a heart attack, 75 people taking the drug still have a heart attack."

The bottom line is you want to reduce the bad (LDL) cholesterol in your blood to cut your risk of having a heart attack. This is most important in people with elevated LDL cholesterol. Changing your diet to include more heart-healthy foods and, if needed, taking cholesterol-reducing drugs called **statins** or bile-binding resins with niacin are your best bets.

4. What is my blood pressure? What can I do to better manage my blood pressure?

High blood pressure (also called **hypertension**) is defined as a systolic pressure (top number) of 140 mm Hg or higher and/or a diastolic pressure (bottom number) of 90 mm Hg or higher. The ideal number combination is less than 120 (systolic, top) over less than 80 (diastolic, bottom).

Hypertension is often underdiagnosed and undertreated. It is a "silent killer" that affects about sixty-five million Americans and one billion people worldwide. High blood pressure directly increases your risk of heart disease and other diseases. It is especially prevalent among African-Americans and people who are elderly, obese, heavy drinkers, and diabetics.

Dr. Kim Allan Williams advises, "African-Americans have more complications from blood pressure probably because they don't have drops in their blood pressure at night."

Statistically, African-Americans have one of the highest rates of hypertension in the world (35 percent). Know your numbers by having your blood pressure checked often. The International Society on Hypertension in Blacks (www.ishib.org) recommends a blood pressure goal of 130/80 or lower.

Healthy lifestyle changes and medicines can help. Cutting salt consumption by eating fewer processed foods and losing your salt shaker will also lower your blood pressure.

Good follow-up questions to ask your doctor include:

- How often should I check my blood pressure?
- Should I buy a home blood pressure monitor?
- Do I need to take blood pressure medicine? If so, for how long and what are the side effects?
- What's my daily salt (sodium) limit?

5. What is my risk of developing diabetes? Or, how can I best manage my diabetes?

Diabetes is deadly. It occurs when the body doesn't produce or properly use insulin, the hormone needed to convert sugar and starches into body energy. The American Diabetes Association states that 23.6 million Americans (7.8 percent) have diabetes. Nearly six million more people are unaware they have the disease.

Doctors test for diabetes or prediabetes with either the fasting plasma glucose (FPG) test or the oral glucose tolerance test (OGTT).

The American Diabetes Association recommends the FPG because it is easier, faster, and less expensive. You can also have a test that shows you what your average blood glucose level has been over the past 10–12 weeks. This test is called a **hemoglobin A1c (or HBA1c)**. Your HBA1c number should be less than 7 percent.

Type 2 diabetes is the most common form. This is a serious but manageable disease. If you are told you have diabetes, prediabetes, or glucose intolerance, be sure you understand your increased risks for heart disease and what actions you need to take, including prescription drugs and lifestyle adjustments. Two large research studies concluded you can prevent or manage Type 2 diabetes with a healthy lifestyle.

6. What physical activity (exercise) do you recommend for me now and later?

Chances are you need more physical activity than you are currently getting. Exercise is vital to good heart health. If you are just recovering from a heart attack, or bypass surgery, or if you are older, or haven't exercised regularly since your college football days, you need to ease into it.

If you are currently in a cardiac rehabilitation program, talk with your doctor or rehabilitation specialist about your progress and any changes he suggests in your exercise routine. Most exercise experts recommend finding a regular physical activity that you enjoy, because you are more likely to continue it long term. Think of it as play instead of work. Exercise doesn't have to be strenuous or boring.

Bill Sonnemaker, MS, an award-winning personal trainer in Atlanta, advises, "If you are coming off a cardiac event, while it's important that you use care and caution, you need aerobic training to put the demand on your system to help your heart."

Ask these additional follow-up questions:

- How much exercise and what types of exercise do you recommend for me?
- Can I play sports? Which ones are best?
- Can I have sex? (See chapter 22).
- What is my target heart rate during exercise? (See chapter 12, Best Question 9.)
- Are there any exercise limitations and precautions?

7. What can I do to quit smoking or drinking too much alcohol?

Ask your doctor for help, advice, and medications if your smoking or drinking habits are contributing to your heart disease. Some heart patients find that their increased stress levels and depression, especially after a cardiac event, contribute to their continued use of tobacco or alcohol even though they want to quit.

Good follow-up questions here are, "What advice do you have about how I can manage my stress levels (or depression)?" "Do you recommend that I take prescription medications to help me?"

Use chapters 18 and 19 for more information and to self-assess your dependency on tobacco or alcohol. Chapter 18 also has specific questions to ask your doctor if you are a smoker.

8. What are my genetic risk factors and what can I do about them?

Maybe you're stuck with heart risk factors that you were born with. Being a man, older, a menopausal woman, or African-American or Native American raises your risk of heart disease. See more at the Centers for Disease Control and Prevention's Web site: www.cdc.gov/genomics/public/famhist.htm.

You are also at increased risk if you have a strong family history of heart disease. This is defined as your grandfather, father, or brother developing heart disease before the age of fifty-five, or your grandmother, mother, or sister developing it before the age of sixty-five.

There are also lesser-known genetic risks, such as a type of genetic high cholesterol called **familial combined hyperlipidemia (FCHL)**, which affects only 1 percent of the population. A severely elevated amount of a chemical called **homocysteine** is a risk marker and can occur rarely as a hereditary disease. Other genetic risks include **HPA-2 Met,** which makes the blood stickier and more likely to clot; **Apo-E4,** a gene linked to a higher risk of heart disease, especially for people who eat the typical high-fat American diet; and **Apo-E2** or **Apo-E3,** both of which don't respond well to lifestyle changes. Another inherited genetic risk is called **Lp(a)** which acts like LDL (bad) cholesterol by increasing your body's tendency to form small clots.

Regardless of your genetic predisposition, adopting the healthy lifestyle changes and/or medications your doctor recommends can help you.

An important follow-up question to ask your doctor is what you need to tell your children about the possibility that they have inherited a risk for heart disease, too. As clinical director of Stanford University's Heart Network Kathy Berra explains, "It's a family affair. Your heart risk factors can be passed on to your son or daughter's heart, too."

9. What am I doing *right* that I should keep on doing or do more of?

Okay, the odds are that even if you've had a heart attack at age forty-two and love deep-fried Oreos, there's something about your health, diet, or weight that you've actually done right up until now. Hearing a small piece of good news in the midst of all the lifestyle changes you're probably facing will be a good morale booster.

There's no sense in stopping your good habits while trying to fix your bad habits. For example, your daily glass of wine or beer may be protecting your heart more than you realize, according to a

2008 Harvard study that found moderate drinking was associated with a lower risk of heart attack.

10. How often should I see you for checkups? How can I communicate with you or your office between appointments if I have questions or concerns?

Be sure to ask these important questions at the end of your office visit, especially if you are just recovering from a heart attack, so you aren't left wondering.

> The Magic Question

What are my other less obvious risks factors?

There are numerous risk factors linked to heart disease that researchers are only starting to understand. For example, a 2008 article in the journal *Circulation* called on experts to study a possible connection between sleep apnea (breathing irregularities during sleep) and cardiovascular disease. In a 2007 study, *JAMA* (the *Journal of the American Medical Association*) reported that heart disease sufferers have twice the risk of bowel cancer as other people. Other studies have concluded coronary artery disease may prematurely dull the brain, air pollution may harm heart attack survivors, and many people overlook leg pain as a warning sign of blocked arteries and the common circulatory problems of **peripheral artery disease (PAD)** where the legs don't get enough blood.

Many doctors won't think to consider your additional "hidden" risk factors, so take the initiative by asking this question.

CONCLUSION

You *can* control your heart disease and prevent another heart attack by living a heart-healthy lifestyle. Family history is not destiny.

Cleveland Clinic's preventive medicine consultant Dr. Caldwell

B. Esselstyn concludes, "Your genes 'load the gun,' but your lifestyle 'pulls the trigger' when it comes to having heart disease and heart attacks."

THE 10 BEST RESOURCES

American Heart Association. "Cardiovascular Conditions." www.ameri canheart.org/presenter.jhtml?identifier=3004349.

American Heart Association. "Heart Attack/Coronary Heart Disease Risk Assessment." www.americanheart.org/presenter.jhtml?identifier=3003499.

Canadian Cardiac Rehabilitation Foundation. "Tips for Your Doctor's Appointment." www.cardiacrehabilitation.ca/documents/doctors_appt.php.

LookAfterYourHeart.com. "Heart Attack Early Warning Signs." www. heart-attack-and-heart-disease.com/Heartattackearlywarningsigns.html.

MedlinePlus. "Heart Diseases: Prevention." www.nlm.nih.gov/medline plus/heartdiseasesprevention.html.

National Cholesterol Education Program. "Risk Assessment Tool for Estimating Your 10-Year Risk of Having a Heart Attack." http://hp2010 .nhlbihin.net/atpiii/calculator.asp?usertype=pub.

National Heart Lung and Blood Institute. "Your Guide to Living Well with Heart Disease." www.nhlbi.nih.gov/health/public/heart/other/your_ guide/living_hd_fs.pdf.

Superko, Robert H., and Laura Tucker. *Before the Heart Attacks: A Revolutionary Approach to Detecting, Preventing, and Even Reversing Heart Disease.* Emmaus, PA: Rodale Press, 2003.

U.S. Food and Drug Administration. "Risk Factors for Cardiovascular Disease." www.fda.gov/hearthealth/riskfactors/riskfactors.html.

Wall Street Journal. "Heart Attacks Across the Globe Are Linked to Nine Risk Factors." August 30, 2004. http://alcohol411.info/HeartAttacks.htm.

CHAPTER 8: THE 10 BEST QUESTIONS
For Women About Heart Health

You can't be brave if you've only had wonderful things
happen to you.

—Mary Tyler Moore

You may be surprised to learn that heart disease is the number one killer of women in the United States. Heart disease takes more women's lives than all other causes combined, including breast cancer. One of every four women dies from heart disease.

Heart disease isn't very sexy. Women are less likely than men to get the appropriate testing to diagnose their heart disease. Women and younger patients are more likely than older men to be sent home from the hospital by mistake or before all commonly recommended tests and procedures are conducted.

Many women (and some doctors) still think that heart disease is a man's disease and that women rarely have heart attacks unless they are old. Since heart disease isn't on many women's radar screens, they often fail to recognize the warning signs of a heart attack and get immediate emergency medical care. This often results in greater heart damage.

The gender gap continues during recovery. Fewer women than men get cardiac rehabilitation or guidance from their doctors on preventive heart care. This may partially explain why fifty thousand more women than men in the United States die from heart disease every year.

There is a growing consensus among heart specialists that heart disease does affect men and women differently, but those differences are only beginning to be understood. Women generally have

THE QUESTION DOCTOR SAYS:

Take charge of mending your own broken heart. Don't worry about upsetting a doctor with your questions. You need his answers. Choose a doctor who welcomes your questions and isn't threatened by your quest for more knowledge and facts.

smaller coronary arteries, which can be more susceptible to plaque buildup and blood clots. Smaller arteries can represent a technical challenge for doctors performing surgeries, angioplasties, or inserting stents.

The following Best Questions assume you are a woman talking to your cardiologist or family doctor after a cardiac event or a diagnosis of heart disease.

>>> THE 10 BEST QUESTIONS
For Women About Heart Health

1. Have I gotten all the appropriate tests, procedures, and treatments I need? Are there any other tests, procedures, or treatments that I need now or later?

The odds are that as a woman you may not have received the full range of tests, procedures, medications, or surgical options that male cardiac patients are offered. This unfortunate gender discrimination in the medical system is especially true if you are an elderly woman. Many women recall having to assertively demand an electrocardiogram to prove their heart attack was happening.

Dr. Sharonne Hayes, director of the Mayo Clinic Women's Heart Clinic, says, "Women tend to be undertreated. For example, there may be an assumption by health care providers that an older woman doesn't want all the trouble of certain treatments."

Treatment options vary widely. A best response is your doctor's thoughtful reconsideration of your medical records and recovery goals rather than a snap answer like, "Of course." Make him think twice about *your* case and avoid mediocre cookie-cutter care.

2. Have these tests or drugs that you are recommending been validated in women? Have my previous test results been interpreted accurately based on my gender?

There are many tests, drugs, and procedures your doctor may recommend for you. When your doctor makes a recommendation, it's appropriate to ask if this test or drug has been proved effective for women in clinical trials.

Ask, "Have gender studies been done on this test/drug? What were the results?" Many heart tests and drugs haven't been as thoroughly researched for women.

Be aware that some tests are less accurate in women, such as the stress electrocardiogram (treadmill test). Estrogen can cause a misinterpretation of the results if the test is not interpreted in a gender-specific manner. Your doctor should prescribe drugs and dosages according to your gender, physical size, and age.

Dr. Hayes advises, "If a treatment hasn't been proven in women, that doesn't automatically mean you shouldn't be on it. It's a good question to ask because it prompts the physician to think more carefully about your care."

3. What are my risk factors for heart disease or another heart attack that I can't control?

Risk factors can be divided between nature and nurture. Natural risk factors are the ones you can't avoid, control, or change. These include a family history of early heart disease for a first-degree relative (before the age of fifty-five for your father or brother and before the age of sixty-five for your mother or sister), certain genetic markers, and being age fifty-five or older and postmenopausal.

Premenopausal women have fewer heart attacks than men. But by the age of seventy-five, the typical risk factors (high blood pressure, elevated cholesterol, etc.) have evened out between men and women.

If you are a diabetic woman, you are at a very high risk for heart disease even at a younger age. Nearly six million American women have been diagnosed with diabetes and nearly three million more are undiagnosed. Diabetes management is possible with weight control, diet, and exercise. Medications for diabetes are often necessary but with a healthy lifestyle you can reduce your dependence on them.

4. What are my risk factors that can be controlled by improving my lifestyle habits? How can I make sure I don't have another heart attack?

Making lifestyle changes is often all that's needed. In fact, the American Heart Association says women can lower their heart disease risk by as much as 82 percent just by leading a healthy lifestyle. Even if you've had a heart attack, you can still reduce the risk of another one.

The most important risk factor within your control is smoking. Dr. Hayes says, "Smoking is such a powerful risk factor that it trumps genetic risk factors." A 2008 study found that women who smoke have heart attacks fourteen years earlier than nonsmoking women. See chapter 18.

Other factors within your control include weight, diet, exercise, alcohol consumption, a quick temper, and reactions to stress.

5. What are my long-term treatment options based on my medical history and risk factors?

Ask your doctor to describe in detail your treatment and surgical options, possible drug side effects, and complementary medicine choices (herbal supplements, yoga for stress reduction, etc.).

There are no quick fixes for heart disease even if you've had an angioplasty or take medications. About 35 percent of women who have had a heart attack will have another one within six years. But experts universally agree that you have more power over your own fate than you might think.

6. What is your best advice about whether I should take hormone replacement therapy (HRT)?

After menopause, your estrogen levels gradually drop along with an increase in LDL ("bad" cholesterol) and a small decrease in HDL ("good" cholesterol). Most doctors now recommend against hormone therapy for postmenopausal women and birth control pills for premenopausal women with a history of heart disease, at least for long-term use.

This recommendation is based on the Heart and Estrogen/Progestin Replacement (HERS) Study that did not find a reduction in heart attacks in women with heart disease who took hormone therapy. The 2008 Women's Health Initiative follow-up report confirmed the health risks of long-term estrogen-progestin hormone therapy for women without a history of heart disease.

This information may change, so make sure you ask your doctor for her latest recommendations. If you are menopausal and have hot flashes or other problems with menopause, ask your doctor for help with nonhormonal therapies.

7. How does my heart disease or heart attack affect my children's and other family members' health? What should I tell my children?

Heart disease can be a family illness. Your heart is your son's and daughter's heart, too. Dr. H. Robert Superko, the executive director of the Center for Genomics and Human Health at Atlanta's St. Joseph's Translational Research Institute, comments, "Women are the medical keepers of the family. Doctors rely on women to enhance compliance and also for access to other family members."

Ask for guidance on talking with your children, especially if you are a heart patient under age sixty-five and of nonwhite descent. Heart disease in young people is more deadly, and it's the biggest killer of young African-American women.

Ask your doctor about your **genetic risk factors,** such as high cholesterol or a tendency toward diabetes or hypertension. Ask if you, your children, or other family members need to be tested for genetic risk factors.

This knowledge can be a lifesaver. Stanford University's Kathy Berra advises telling children, "When there's heart disease in your family, it's not a noose around your neck. Think of it as an opportunity. You *can* make positive lifestyle changes and live longer than your relatives."

8. When can I start cardiac rehabilitation? What specific recommendations do you have for my cardiac rehab program?

The experts interviewed for this book unanimously sang the praises of cardiac rehab, especially for women. Dr. Hayes advises adamantly, "If you are offered cardiac rehab, do it! If you aren't offered rehab, ask for it!"

Cardiologist Dr. Mimi Guarneri, medical director of the Scripps Center for Integrative Medicine in La Jolla, California, agrees: "Women tend to take care of everyone else and not themselves. The biggest lesson for women is that they have to start putting themselves first by going to cardiac rehab."

Cardiac rehab has physical benefits, has social and emotional support systems, and helps you to internalize healthier eating and exercise habits for the rest of your life. Don't take no for an answer.

Most insurance providers cover it. If you have logistical barriers (live in a rural location, are not permitted to drive, etc.), ask about home-based, phone-based, and long-distance versions of cardiac rehab. See chapter 12.

9. What symptoms are warning signs of a heart attack in women? What special precautions should I take?

Heart attack symptoms in women are not necessarily the same as for men, who often say a heart attack feels like an elephant stomping on their chest. Women also experience chest pain, but their symptoms might include one or more of these more subtle factors:

- Neck, jaw, and shoulder pain
- Abdominal pain
- Nausea
- Vomiting
- Extreme fatigue
- Shortness of breath
- Trouble sleeping

Dr. Jessica Black, a naturopathic physician in McMinnville, Oregon, advises, "Women often have reoccurring symptoms for a while before the heart attack comes. Sometimes women aren't aware because their symptoms aren't as dramatic as men's symptoms are."

Lisa M. Tate, CEO of WomenHeart, says, "You hear about the Tim Russerts of the world dying at fifty, but heart disease is often not as dramatic for women. Women don't perceive themselves to be at risk for heart disease, when in fact they are."

When having a heart attack, some women encounter unacceptable delays from medical personnel or seek medical care later than men. Silent heart attacks are more common in women. Ask your doctor for suggestions and precautions.

10. What symptoms are serious enough that I should call you? What should I do if I think I'm having a heart attack?

Rather than second guessing when to call your doctor or being reluctant to call because you don't want to bother her, get the straight facts now based on your personal cardiac history. *If you think you are having a heart attack, call 911, not the doctor's office.* Every minute counts in an emergency.

> The Magic Question

What's the latest thing you have read or learned about women and heart disease?

This is a repeated Magic Question from chapter 4, this time with a "woman" angle. As a woman with heart disease, it's absolutely vital you have a doctor who knows the latest research on how heart disease affects women differently from men. Women are more likely than men to have misleading or inaccurate test results.

For example, a ten-year study published in 2006, called the WISE Study (Women's Ischemia Syndrome Evaluation), concluded that diagnostic angiograms for some women indicating clear arteries may be incorrect for as many as three million women. Some women have a condition called **coronary microvascular syndrome,** where cholesterol plaque that accumulates in very small arteries doesn't show up on the standard angiogram. These women rarely get the proper treatment and remain at high risk for having a heart attack. If your doctor has heard of the WISE study or seems confidently aware of other key trends and studies for women cardiac patients, consider her a keeper.

CONCLUSION

This is no time to be passive. As a woman, you may have taken care of all the other people in your life—your children, your partner, perhaps your aging parents. Consider your heart disease or heart attack your wakeup call to look out for "Number One" now.

Be proactive. Get into cardiac rehab. Ask the Best Questions and any other questions important to you. Stick to your guns and learn as much as you can about heart disease and risk factors within your control.

Dr. Caela Farren, a management consultant in Virginia, recalls her 2004 heart attack: "My biggest learning is that you have to take charge of your own situation and be your own best advocate. Beforehand, I knew nothing about this because I just assumed it would never happen to me."

THE 10 BEST RESOURCES

American Heart Association. "Women and Cardiovascular Disease." www .americanheart.org/presenter.jhtml?identifier=1200011.

Boston Women's Health Book Collective and Judy Norsigian. *Our Bodies, Ourselves: A New Edition for a New Era,* 4th ed. New York: Touchstone, 2005.

Cleveland Clinic. "Women's Heart: Move It!" http://my.clevelandclinic .org/newsletters/heart/2007summer/moveit.aspx.

Gaudet, Tracy, Paula Spencer, and Andrew Weil. *Consciously Female: How to Listen to Your Body and Your Soul for a Lifetime of Healthier Living.* New York: Bantam, 2004.

Goldberg, Nieca. *The Women's Healthy Heart Program: Lifesaving Strategies for Preventing and Healing Heart Disease.* New York: Ballantine Books, 2006.

Medline Plus. "Heart Disease in Women." www.nlm.nih.gov/medline plus/heartdiseaseinwomen.html.

National Institutes of Health. "WISE Study of Women and Heart Disease Yields Important Findings on a Frequently Undiagnosed Coronary Syndrome." www.nih.gov/news/pr/jan2006/nhlbi-31.htm.

Northrup, Christine. *Women's Bodies, Women's Wisdom: Creating Physical and Emotional Health and Healing.* New York: Bantam, 2006.

WebMD. "The Heart Truth for Women: It's Ageless." www.webmd.com/heart-disease/womens-risk.

WomenHeart. "Women and Heart Disease Fact Sheet." www.women heart.org/information/women_and_heart_disease_fact_sheet.asp.

PART II

Choosing Treatments

Surviving a heart attack or discovering you have heart disease is terribly confusing and upsetting. You suddenly find you must make important decisions about health care, but it's hard to know all the facts or where to turn for advice. Most people feel overwhelmed, depressed, or panicked.

Former surgeon general Dr. C. Everett Koop has firsthand experience, too. He says, "I nearly died from cardiac failure. I was essentially dead and was resuscitated. I had my heart operated on and now I'm in the best cardiac shape I've been in in a long, long time. It's given me a new lease on life."

There are as many uniquely personal reactions to a heart attack as there are choices of treatments. Not everyone wants to do a lot of research or become a walking encyclopedia on heart disease, yet others wouldn't have it any other way. Some people reach out for aggressive therapies and to dozens of people for comfort and advice, whereas others choose conservative treatments and prefer privacy.

The 10 Best Questions in this section will help to strengthen your decision-making muscles. Because heart disease is basically incurable, you and your doctor will look for the best ways to prevent further damage with a combination of surgeries, interventional procedures, drugs, alternative therapies, and heart-healthy lifestyle changes.

Sorting through your personal priorities and learning about your treatment options will bring you a greater measure of comfort and self-confidence. Chapter 9 suggests what to ask about heart medications. In chapters 10 and 11, you'll learn what to ask about proposed heart surgeries and when choosing a hospital. Cardiac rehabilitation, a key component in mending your broken heart, is discussed in chapter 12. If you want to know more about alternative therapies (also called complementary or integrative medicine) and how to avoid being ripped off by a scam artist, see chapter 13.

The Question Doctor sincerely hopes the following Best Questions on treatment choices will ease your journey. Your doctor may be an authority on medicine, but you are the world's foremost expert on yourself.

CHAPTER 9: THE 10 BEST QUESTIONS

To Ask About Heart Medications

> It is easy to get a thousand prescriptions but hard to get one single remedy.
>
> —Chinese proverb

Heart disease medications reduce the symptoms associated with coronary artery disease (CAD), prevent a heart attack or heart failure, and slow the progression of heart disease. Your doctor may prescribe a variety of heart drugs to lower your cholesterol or blood pressure, to ease chest pains (called angina), or for abnormal heart rhythms (called arrhythmias).

The combination of medications will be based on your symptoms and medical history. It's in your best interest to know the names of these medications, their benefits, potential side effects, and when to talk to your doctor about your prescriptions. If you've had a heart attack or been diagnosed with severe heart disease, you will need to take medication for the rest of your life, so you need to understand its long-term effects, too.

Ask your doctor the following Best Questions about her recommendations for prescription heart drugs, other medications, and

---

THE QUESTION DOCTOR SAYS:

Consider taking a tape recorder or a notepad with you when you see your doctor. Many people are intimidated by discussions about complex drugs with unfamiliar names. You can listen to the tape later or review your notes without the additional pressure of being face-to-face with the doctor. Ask your doctor to write down both the generic and brand names for any drugs she prescribes for you.

your treatments in general. Be sure to check with your insurance provider or Medicare about payment coverage details.

>>> THE 10 BEST QUESTIONS
To Ask About Heart Medications

1. What drugs do you recommend I take for my heart disease? Why? Please explain how these drugs work.

There are many types and combinations of medications to treat heart disease (coronary artery disease) and related conditions. Depending on the type and severity of your heart problem and the other medical conditions you have, your doctor can choose from a wide range of possible medications.

To simplify things, Kathy Berra says, "The most important drugs are the ABCs: A is for aspirin and ACE (angiotensin-converting enzyme) inhibitors, B is for beta blockers, and C stands for cholesterol-lowering and calcium channel blockers."

Use this question to open a dialogue with your doctor about the best treatment combination for you. The best answer to the "why?" question will be a full explanation that gives you the sense that your doctor has put thought into your personal case and isn't just giving you the same drugs she routinely prescribes for most heart patients.

While you need to trust your doctor, the savviest patients remain slightly skeptical. No one profits when you eat your vegetables or go to the gym, but both drug companies and some doctors earn money from prescriptions.

Dr. H. Robert Superko, executive director of the Center for Genomics and Human Health at St. Joseph's Translational Research Institute in Atlanta, explains, "When the statin drugs came out, they were very low risk, effective, and have made billions of dollars for drug companies. . . . You can have a profound effect on stopping cardiovascular disease in its tracks, but it's not by statins alone. Niacin plus a statin has been the combination selected by National Institutes of Health doctors for heart disease regression studies."

Another potential danger is suggested by Dr. Larry F. Hamm, president of the American Association of Cardiovascular and Pulmonary Rehabilitation and a cardiac rehabilitation specialist at The George Washington University. He says, "In reality, sometimes doctors are so focused on drugs that they may not refer you to cardiac rehabilitation in a timely fashion."

2. What percentage of improvement can I reasonably expect from this drug?

As you weigh the potential risks and benefits of taking any drug, hearing about the positive effects as a percentage may help clarify the facts. Ask your doctor to talk in specific terms, such as the average percentage of improvement for clogged arteries or reduced angina symptoms (chest pains).

No doctor can predict with absolute certainty how well a medication will help you, but this discussion establishes realistic expectations. Another big variable is your willingness to adopt healthier eating and exercise habits. Be sure your doctor explains your personal potential benefits and not just national averages.

3. How will you know if this drug is working well?

It's equally important to understand the details of how your doctor plans to assess and monitor a proposed drug's effectiveness over time, especially since heart disease is a silent and invisible killer.

Also ask, "How often will I need to make follow-up visits to the doctor's office or for laboratory tests?" and "How long will I have to take this drug for it to be effective?"

4. What short-term side effects are possible? Long-term side effects? Are there any side effects that may not go away?

Get the specifics on both short-term and long-term side effects. Be sure your doctor addresses this question for your specific case and not just with data from clinical trials or general studies.

Don't let your doctor gloss over his answer to this question. Double-check his response by searching the Internet for this medication by its generic and brand names. And don't forget to ask about potential permanent side effects and toxicity—a great question that few people think to ask.

5. How will you (the doctor) help me to manage any side effects?

This question will help you to learn more about side effects and if there are ways to lessen their impact on your health and well-being. For example, if you experience stomach upset, which is common with some heart medications, there may be simple over-the-counter remedies or another prescription to help control this problem.

6. What can I do to minimize the side effects and stay healthy?

Asking this question will help you feel like you are more in control of your own health. This question also implies that you and your doctor are a team, with both of you actively involved in your well-being.

Your doctor will probably also discuss alternative treatments, diet, and exercise as healthy lifestyle strategies to improve your heart health. See part three for more on healthy lifestyles.

7. What, if any, restrictions will there be on my normal activities while I'm taking this drug?

Be sure you understand if there are any prohibitions on foods, other drugs, alcohol use, or any additional considerations you should know in advance. This is especially true if you still live a normal and active lifestyle, including travel, work, sex, sports, and outdoor activities.

8. What should I do if I miss a dose of my medicine?

Use your doctor's answer to solve any mysteries about whether you should double up or not in order to compensate for missed dosages. Keep in mind that it's generally not a good idea to double up on dosages, especially for medications like digitalis or Coumadin (warfarin). Call your doctor later if you need further clarification.

9. What changes in my symptoms are serious enough for me to call you?

Find out the specifics, such as chest pains or shortness of breath. Ask your doctor to review with you the warning signs of a heart attack, especially if you are a woman. Women typically have less dramatic or obvious symptoms.

Many people hesitate to call their doctors for fear of "bothering" them or overreacting to new symptoms. Let your doctor's response guide you to a better-informed decision that might even save your life.

10. What is my overall treatment plan?

In addition to discussing specific drugs, find out the big picture for your long-term heart care and treatment. An overall treatment plan may include more tests or an angioplasty to check for and treat any blockages.

Ask if the proposed treatment options will interfere with your other medications or will include lifestyle changes (more exercise, etc.). Be sure your doctor's plan specifies heart medications and drugs for your other medical conditions. Ask specifically if you should take an aspirin every day and its dosage. Many doctors recommend aspirin for most people with known coronary or vascular disease.

Finally, discuss with your doctor if you must take this drug for the rest of your life or at which point you may no longer need it.

❯ The Magic Question

Are there less expensive medications for my heart condition? Is there a generic version of this drug that is just as effective and cheaper?

Many people with heart disease, especially if they are heart attack survivors, have to take certain heart medications for the rest of their lives. This is an important question to ask now at the onset of your heart treatment that could potentially save you hundreds or thousands of dollars.

Not all generic drugs are the same high-grade quality as their brand-name counterparts, so find out the specifics on drugs your doctor has recommended.

Seniors are the largest consumers of the $200 billion per year prescription drug industry in America. Drug companies spend enormous amounts of money and effort to convince doctors and older patients that their products are a worthy investment. With a diagnosis as frightening as heart disease, you may not stop to consider, "What exactly am I putting in my body?" "Is it worth it?" "Is this drug a good value for my money?"

CARDIAC MEDICATIONS: A PRIMER

Here are the most commonly prescribed types of drugs and what they are used for. Many people with heart disease also take various antibiotics, antidepressants, anti-inflammatories, fibric acids, niacin (nicotinic acid), and supplements and vitamins.

> **Anticoagulants** are blood thinners that prevent the clotting associated with coronary artery disease. If you have atrial fibrillation (an irregular heart rhythm), you have a high risk of a blood clot forming in your heart that can travel to your brain and cause a stroke. Anticoagulants are closely monitored to prevent excessive bleeding.

> **Antiplatelets** keep the blood platelets from sticking together. They help prevent heart attacks, angina, and other cardiovascular diseases. Aspirin and clopidogrel (Plavix) are common examples.

> **ACE inhibitors (angiotensin-converting enzyme)** and **angiotensin II receptor blockers (ARBs)** prevent heart enlargement after a heart attack and help improve blood flow, high blood pressure, and heart failure.

> **Beta blockers** decrease heart rate and cardiac output, lower blood pressure, prevent heart attacks, and treat angina and arrhythmias.

> **Calcium channel blockers** interrupt the movement of calcium into the heart and treat high blood pressure, angina, and arrhythmias.

> **Diuretics (water pills)** help the body to get rid of excess fluids, lower blood pressure, and reduce swelling (edema).

> **Digitalis** helps to relieve heart failure and slows the high heart rate associated with arrhythmias such as atrial fibrillation.

> **Vasodilators (nitroglycerin pills or nitrates)** relax blood vessels, increase blood and oxygen to the heart, and help to ease angina.

> **Lipid-lowering agents (statins)** lower LDL ("bad") cholesterol, raise HDL ("good") cholesterol, and lower triglyceride levels. Nearly all heart attack survivors benefit from long-term lipid therapy.

CONCLUSION

Use your doctor's advice and answers to make a better-informed decision about the drugs that he is recommending for your heart treatment. If you are still unsure about what to do, ask your doctor this follow-up question: "If you were making this decision for your parent or a loved one with heart disease like mine, what would you do?"

Consider your personal priorities and financial situation as you ask *yourself* these two questions: "Are these drugs cost effective for me?" "Will they improve my quality of life?"

Everyone's heart disease and situation is different, so there is no right or wrong answer. Some people are happy for any slight improvement, while others dismiss small improvements as insufficient to justify the cost or hassle. Your quality-of-life issues are an important consideration as you evaluate what's best for you.

THE 10 BEST RESOURCES

American Heart Association. "Cardiac Medications At-A-Glance." www .americanheart.org/presenter.jhtml?identifier=3038846.

American Heart Association. "How Do I Manage My Medicines?" www .americanheart.org/downloadable/heart/1196285659399ManageMedi cine.pdf.

Drugs.com. "Heart Disease Medications." www.drugs.com/condition/ heart-disease.html.

Food and Drug Administration. "Electronic Orange Book: Approved Drug Products with Therapeutic Equivalence Evaluations." www.fda.gov/ cder/ob/default.htm.

Food and Drug Administration. "Information About the Products We Regulate." www.fda.gov/cder/drug/default.htm.

HealthCentral. "Heart Disease Drug Information." www.healthcentral .com/heart-disease/drugs.html.

IGuard.org. "Search Drugs." http://iguard.org.

Medline Plus. "Drugs, Supplements, and Herbal Information." (Search by drug name.) www.nlm.nih.gov/medlineplus/druginformation.html.

National Heart Lung and Blood Institute. "Heart Disease and Medications." www.nhlbi.nih.gov/actintime/hdm/hdm.htm.

WebMD. "Heart Disease: How to Take Your Heart Medication." www .webmd.com/heart-disease/guide/how-take-medication.

CHAPTER 10: THE 10 BEST QUESTIONS
About Heart Surgery

I got the bill for my surgery. Now I know what those
doctors were wearing masks for.
> —James H. Boren, humorist and author

Unless you had emergency heart surgery immediately following a heart attack, you'll probably have time to discuss your surgical options and questions. A heart attack
is one emergency with no time for questions. But many heart patients can make less rushed decisions about their treatment options,
which often include a combination of surgeries, cardiac catheterizations (coronary angioplasties and stenting), medications, and lifestyle changes.

Thousands of people have heart surgery every day. You owe it to
yourself to understand why your doctor is recommending it for you,
other treatment options, and the potential risks and benefits. You
may also want a second opinion. See chapter 6.

Some questions about surgery are obvious, while other questions may not have occurred to you. The following Best Questions
will help you make a well-educated decision and guide your conversations with your surgeon or cardiologist.

>>> THE 10 BEST QUESTIONS
About Heart Surgery

1. What are my other treatment options (if any) instead of this surgery? If none, please explain why you recommend this surgery for me.

If you don't ask this question now, you may never know. Dr. Timothy J. Gardner, president of the American Heart Association, says,

"For patients without urgent needs, the treatment options are broader. Catheterization and stenting may not be among their best options. Medical treatment may be better. For these patients, the careful consideration of options with the doctor is especially called for."

Dr. Sharonne Hayes, director of the Mayo Clinic Women's Heart Clinic, advises, "Keep in mind that cardiac surgeons are going to tell you they want to operate. Cardiologists are going to recommend either medical therapy or interventions like stents. You need to visit with both and weigh your options."

Likewise, Kathy Berra, MSN, clinical director of Stanford University's Heart Network says, "If someone told me I needed open heart surgery, I would get a second opinion, no question. If the surgeon doesn't want you to get a second opinion, I wouldn't go to that doctor." (See chapter 6 on second opinions.)

2. Which type of heart surgery do you recommend for me? Why? What are the specific objectives and benefits of this surgery in my case?

There are many types and reasons for heart surgeries. For example, surgeries can bypass or widen blocked arteries, repair or replace heart valves, implant devices to regulate heart rhythms, boost the heart's pumping power, prevent sudden cardiac death, and repair **aneurysms** (bulges in the aorta).

Two common surgeries are **coronary artery bypass graft (CABG)** and **coronary angioplasty** (or **balloon angioplasty** with or without **coronary artery stenting**). In CABG surgery, a patient's leg vein or chest artery is used to create a new route around a blockage. Surgeons often use your own arteries (mammary arteries) that generally last longer than vein grafts. Ask your surgeon which kind he plans to use.

Coronary angioplasty treats atherosclerosis by widening an obstructed blood vessel using a balloon catheter. This is technically considered an interventional procedure rather than a surgery, is minimally invasive, and is also called a **percutaneous coronary intervention.**

A small mesh tube called a **stent** is sometimes inserted into the blood vessel to keep it open. There's controversy among doctors about using stents, especially drug-covered versus bare stents. Ask your doctor about his views on this prior to your procedure.

Other types of heart surgeries include the following:

- **Open-heart surgery** is any kind of heart surgery where the chest wall is opened to operate on the heart. It is used to bypass blocked heart arteries, repair or replace heart valves, fix **atrial fibrillation** (abnormal heart rhythm), and for heart transplants.
- **Heart transplantation** is the replacement of a patient's diseased or injured heart with a healthy donor heart. It is usually recommended only for end-stage heart failure and after all other possible treatments have failed.
- **Balloon valvuloplasty,** also called **percutaneous balloon valvuloplasty,** is a surgical procedure to open a narrowed heart valve, a condition called **stenosis,** in order to improve valve function and blood flow.
- Implantation of a **pacemaker** or **defibrillator** helps the heart to beat more regularly and correct life-threatening irregular rhythms such as **ventricular fibrillation** or **ventricular tachycardia.**

Good follow-up questions include: "How long can I expect relief?" "How long will my heart's functioning be better?" "What will happen if this surgery isn't successful?"

Kathy Berra warns, "For a lot of people, their surgeon will come in and say, 'You're all fixed now.' Well, baloney. They may have fixed the big blockages, but it's the little ones that are going to rupture and kill you. Like Tim Russert."

3. Am I a candidate for minimally invasive surgery? Why or why not?

Minimally invasive heart surgery means the surgeon cuts smaller or fewer incisions and uses tiny cameras or robot-assisted arms. Its advantages include less blood loss and trauma to your body, smaller scars, and shorter recovery time.

Off-pump heart surgery (also called **beating heart surgery**) is similar to open-heart surgery except you aren't connected to a heart–lung bypass machine. This results in fewer complications and a faster recovery.

Minimally invasive coronary artery bypass surgeries (also called **off-pump coronary artery bypass surgery** and **minimally invasive direct coronary artery bypass surgery**) have been recently developed that forego a heart–lung machine and speed recovery.

4. How many times did you perform this recommended surgery during the past year? What is your personal preference for surgery over other options? What is your reoperation rate?

In general, the more surgeries under a surgeon's belt the better. See chapter 4 for more on surgeons' credentials.

A difficult problem when seeking a surgeon's advice is trying to understand his personal biases for surgery over the full spectrum of your other treatment options. Just like the differences between Republicans and Democrats, everyone has biases.

For example, if your surgeon has a strong bias for doing angioplasties, he may routinely recommend them without fully considering medications and/or lifestyle alternatives. Avoid a doctor who knows or performs only a small handful of treatments.

There's also a fear factor. Many heart attack survivors and their families are so afraid of the "next big one" that they choose the most aggressive surgery possible without fully considering their other options. However, a study described in the July 2008 issue of *Consumer Reports* warned that the patients who were treated most aggressively were at an increased risk of infections, surgical complications, and medical errors.

The results of a landmark 2007 study called COURAGE Trial (Clinical Outcomes Utilizing Revascularization and Aggressive Drug Evaluation) found that patients who had angioplasties and stents plus intensive lifestyle changes and medications did no better than comparable patients who received drug therapy only. The president of the American Heart Association, Dr. Timothy J. Gardner, comments, "The study showed that although the treatment with stents helped to reduce chest pains, it did not provide any benefits for survival at two, five, or ten years."

The reoperation rate is how many patients a surgeon has to operate on again for various reasons, some not totally within her control. The national average is 5 percent. Most surgeons will know their number.

5. Please describe this surgery and how long it will take. Where will it be performed? When can my family see me?

Ask your doctor or surgeon to explain it in simple terms including the exact procedure, location, how many hours, and when your family can see you afterward. Surgeons are required to ask you if you fully understand what's going to happen during the surgery.

> **THE QUESTION DOCTOR SAYS:**
>
> Be sure to ask any other questions you feel are important to understanding your surgery. Don't be intimidated by the surgeon. Surgeons' skills as explainers and listeners vary widely. If you are confused, the surgeon hasn't explained it well enough. Period. It's *not* a reflection on you or your intelligence.

6. What are the short-term and long-term risks for this surgery? Will there be any likely long-term changes from this surgery that won't go away?

The most common risks of heart surgery include infection, fever, bleeding, a reaction to medicines, irregular heartbeats, and rarely death. Blood clots sometimes form when a heart-lung bypass machine is used. Most people are uncomfortable for the first few days after surgery. You are likely to have some postsurgical pain. Ask about getting pain relief before you need it.

It's reasonable to ask the doctor for specific estimates or percentages of benefits and risks. Surgeries will have an absolute short-term risk in percentages, like 2 percent. Catheterizations have a slightly lower risk than other procedures. The other important piece of information concerns the risk over time if you don't have this surgery.

Your surgeon's answer should include a thorough explanation of why the benefits of having the recommended surgery outweigh the risks in your case. Don't skip the last part of this question about long-term impact.

7. Who will do the actual surgery? Will you have other doctors or medical students who will assist in a major way? Do I have any choice in this matter?

You want to know who's holding the knives while you're asleep. Some surgeons have assistants or interns take over portions of their surgeries, especially at teaching hospitals associated with medical schools. If you are concerned, ask this follow-up question: "Would you allow a member of your family to be operated on by this person?"

8. What will happen after my surgery?

The amount of time you will be in the hospital depends on the type of surgery you are having. You will be encouraged to get out of bed and move around quickly to speed your recovery.

Ask these follow-up questions as well: "What can I expect during my immediate recovery?" "How long will I be in the hospital?" "Who will be responsible for my care while I'm in the hospital?"

Make sure you know exactly who will be in charge of your care while you are in the hospital. If your surgeon has partners, will they make the hospital rounds instead of your surgeon? How can you reach your surgeon if you have questions? Who will prescribe painkillers for you? Unclear post-op communications can be a great source of patient frustration.

9. How long will the healing take? When can I return to work and my daily routines? Drive? Exercise? Have sex? Will I need someone to help me after I leave the hospital?

Again, your surgeon's answers will vary depending on the surgery and your general health and age. After surgery, expect to hear how to care for yourself.

You may need follow-up medical care, lifestyle changes, medicines, and/or cardiac rehabilitation. Don't be embarrassed to ask personal questions about sex or bodily functions. Follow your surgeon's advice and schedule for returning to normal activities.

10. What is the most probable outcome from this surgery? How likely is it that this surgery will reduce my chest pains or heart risks?

There are no absolute guarantees on surgical outcomes. The ideal answer describes measurable benefits that include taking long-term benefits into account, not just short-term improvements.

› The Magic Question

How long has the operating room team worked together?

A good surgeon typically works with the same few anesthesiologists, nurses, and medical assistants. Of course, there are some personnel changes that are unavoidable. But the longer and more frequently a surgical team has worked together, the better it can work together in case of an emergency or unexpected event.

It's like a football, basketball, or soccer team. There might be star players on the team—a star surgeon, just like a star quarterback—but if they haven't practiced together, they aren't going to the championship playoffs.

Getting a seasoned surgical team may not be an option for you or even a deal breaker, but it's nice if you can get it. And it's probably something that never occurred to you to ask about until now.

CONCLUSION

Heart disease and its treatments are complex. But it's possible to understand your surgery in simple terms if you ask your doctors the right questions.

The results of heart surgery are often excellent. But never forget that the final decision is yours.

THE 10 BEST RESOURCES

American Heart Association. "How Can I Prepare for Heart Surgery?" www.americanheart.org/downloadable/heart/1196353410728Prepare HeartSurgery.pdf.

American Heart Association. "Surgery and Other Medical Procedures." www.americanheart.org/presenter.jhtml?identifier=123.

American Heart Association. "What Happens After Heart Surgery?" www.americanheart.org/downloadable/heart/119626811852451%20 WhtHppnsAftrHrtSrgry%209_07.pdf.

American Heart Association. "What Is Coronary Angioplasty?" www .americanheart.org/downloadable/heart/119626700426849%2What IsCoronaryAngioplasty_9-07.pdf.

British Heart Foundation. "Having Heart Surgery." www.bhf.org.uk/ publications.aspx.

Cleveland Clinic. "Surgery for Heart Failure." http://my.clevelandclinic .org/heart/disorders/heartfailure/hf_surgery.aspx.

Encyclopedia of Surgery. "A Guide for Patients and Caregivers." (Search term "heart surgery.") www.surgeryencyclopedia.com/index.html.

MedlinePlus. "Heart Surgery." www.nlm.nih.gov/medlineplus/heartsurgery .html.

MSN Health & Fitness. "10 Questions You Must Ask Your Doctor." http:// health.msn.com/health-topics/articlepage.aspx?cp-documetid=100182331.

National Heart Lung and Blood Institute. "Types of Heart Surgery." www .nhlbi.nih.gov/health/dci/Diseases/hs/hs_types.html.

CHAPTER 11: THE 10 BEST QUESTIONS
For Choosing a Hospital

A hospital bed is a parked taxi with the meter running.
—Groucho Marx

The prospect of your upcoming heart surgery or procedure is scary enough without worrying about possible hospital infections or adverse drug reactions as frequently reported in medical journals and the national media. This chapter addresses nonemergency hospitalization situations—that is, not when a heart attack or unstable angina is in progress. In emergency cases, there's rarely time for questions and you may not be fully alert.

If your doctor has told you that you need surgery or a procedure done at a hospital and it is not urgent, your next job is to find the very best hospital. Yes, this is yet one more decision in the midst of information overload and emotional turmoil. But if you aren't restricted by your choice of doctors or health insurance coverage, this can be a potentially important—and even lifesaving—decision.

You may choose simply to go to the hospital where your doctor has operating privileges or where you were admitted for your heart attack. If you have chosen your cardiologist and surgeon well and have only a short hospital stay after your surgery, there may be nothing wrong with this choice. Your hospital choices may also be limited by your geographical location, insurance plan, or travel costs.

However, if you do have hospital choices or want the extra assurance of researching the quality of a hospital, ask your doctor or hospital administrators the following Best Questions. Use the second set of Best Questions as assessment questions to ask yourself when you tour a hospital prior to admittance.

THE QUESTION DOCTOR SAYS:

Being an informed patient is your best protection against medical errors and infections. Don't let doctors or nurses brush aside your questions. Overcome your reluctance to speak up. Remain firmly polite as you persevere through your list of questions. Your life may depend on it.

>>> THE 10 BEST QUESTIONS
For Choosing a Hospital

1. Does this hospital provide the specialties and services that will best meet my specific needs for my heart surgery or procedure?

What matters the most is this hospital's track record in heart surgery and follow-up cardiac care. You want a hospital that does lots and lots of heart surgeries routinely at least every week, if not every day.

There's safety in numbers when it comes to surgeries. Keep in mind that smaller hospitals will naturally have fewer surgeries, so ask for percentages to help you put the numbers into proper perspective. A 2006 study concluded that high-volume hospitals have better survival rates.

Kathy Berra advises, "Call the hospital or get from the American Hospital Association their data on how your hospital measures against national standards."

2. Is this a teaching hospital?

A teaching hospital affiliated with a university medical school is a good idea if you have a complicated surgery. Dr. Paul Schyve, a vice president at The Joint Commission, the premier hospital accreditation organization in the United States, says, "Safety science tells us that the more complex the treatment, the more different players that are involved, and the more steps in the process, the greater the likelihood of something going wrong."

In general, teaching hospitals stay more current on cardiac surgical procedures, techniques, and medications. You may have to balance this advantage with the likelihood of there being hoards of hovering interns just like on the television show *Grey's Anatomy.*

3. What is this hospital's accreditation status?

Hospitals' accreditation status can shift up or down over time. Find out if your prospective hospital has a history of conditional accreditations, or even worse, has had a "preliminary denial of accreditation."

The Joint Commission sends out its inspectors at least every three years. If you drill down on their Web site (www.jointcommission.org), you can find information on a hospital's accreditation and standardized measures for surgical care and performance.

Another reliable source of information is HealthGrades, Inc. (www.healthgrades.com). It offers comprehensive reports on hospital ratings, costs, patient volume, and patient safety for a small fee. Its Web site also offers free restaurant-style hospital ratings (one to five stars).

4. Does this hospital appear to be clean?

Cleanliness doesn't guarantee that a hospital has good internal procedures to control infections, but dirty bathrooms are red flags for potential trouble. Consider the sobering statistic that more people die from hospital-acquired infections every year than all accidents and homicides combined.

If the hospital appears dirty, don't go there. Period. The following 10 Best Questions for a hospital tour will help you make this assessment.

5. What procedures are in place for patient safety and infection control?

Ask this question even if the hospital looks and smells clean. Statistically, you have a one in twenty chance of getting an infection during your hospital stay. Approximately two million people develop an infection while in the hospital every year. About ninety thousand Americans die from hospital-acquired infections at an annual cost of $1 billion.

Ask if this hospital has an infection consultant or an infection-control team responsible for making frequent cleanliness checks. Does the hospital isolate high-risk patients? What does the hospital do to protect patients against the new "superbugs," such as antibiotic methicillin-resistant *Staphylococcus aureus* (MRSA) and others, at near epidemic levels in some locations? Researchers found that improved infection practices can reduce the rate of in-hospital infection by up to 70 percent.

The good news is that you can protect yourself during your hospital stay by asking the medical staff two simple questions:

1. Did you just wash your hands?
2. What's my name?

Even if it seems silly, ask every medical person who touches you (yes, even your doctor) if he has just washed his hands. It might sound like something your mother would nag about, but this simple question is a proven lifesaver.

Ask the medical staff to identify you by name to ensure that they are giving you the right drug or treatment. Know the names of your medications. Most hospital mistakes are preventable. Being an assertive patient may save your life.

6. Who will have the primary responsibility for my care while I'm in the hospital? Who will communicate with me, my family, and other members of my medical team?

One of patients' most common complaints is that no one seems to be the central person in charge of their care. This becomes crucial if you need more pain meds, have a problem drain, or are waiting to go home.

Ask this question of both your cardiologist and surgeon before checking into the hospital. You may see several different doctors in the hospital due to their schedule of rotating rounds.

The second question is equally important. Many doctors don't communicate well with one another. Dr. Paul Schyve of The Joint Commission says, "We've discovered that the most common root cause for medical errors on the individual level is communication breakdown."

Make sure your family understands in advance how and when they will be told about the outcome of your surgery.

7. What are my rights and responsibilities as a patient and how will you let me know about them?

It is useful to know your rights as a patient. Every hospital should notify patients about informed consent, privacy during physical examinations, and the right to refuse participation in hospital research experiments.

Ensuring patient satisfaction is not rocket science. Some hospitals have a patient representative or ombudsman department that you can call.

8. How conveniently located is this hospital for me and my visitors?

It makes sense to choose the hospital that's most convenient to where you live, especially if you expect visitors. Just knowing you'll be on familiar turf can boost your morale to handle your upcoming surgery.

Being hometown centered can also reaffirm the importance of being treated at a religiously affiliated hospital or the same facility you've used since childhood. Other patients want to control their visitors. Dr. Rebecca Allison, a Phoenix cardiologist, comments on the needs of same-sex couples: "Some hospitals may refuse to involve the partner or not allow the partner equal visiting rights despite the patient's careful planning for this event."

Before you pack your slippers and head off to your hometown hospital, just make sure you aren't unconsciously sacrificing quality for convenience.

9. Will my insurance cover the costs at this hospital?

Check with both the hospital and your health insurance provider prior to admittance to determine what percentage of your hospital stay will be paid for. Ask the hospital if it has a written description of its services and fees. Check on available resources if you need financial assistance. A hospital-based social worker can help you with information, resources, and advice. See also chapter 24.

10. How will you (the hospital staff) prepare me for leaving the hospital?

Once your surgery is over, it's not the end of the story. Ask if you or your caregiver will be given a written detailed discharge plan. Confirm that a copy of your medical records will go to your primary care doctor.

A good look at a hospital's discharge procedures can help you assess this hospital's overall quality. In the actual discharge plan, look for nitty-gritty instructions, such as how to change your bandages and medication schedules after you get home. Ask if you can drive, have sex, and when you can resume your other normal activities.

The George Washington University's visiting professor and cardiac rehabilitation specialist Dr. Larry Hamm says, "Patients need to make sure they have a firm plan in place when they leave the hospital. This is very important, because communicating with the health care professionals is much harder after you've been discharged. Don't be shy about asking questions, even a couple of times."

❯ The Magic Question

Does this hospital have social workers to assist me? How accessible are they?

Social workers help patients and their families find emotional, social, clinical, physical, and financial support services. The presence of social workers on the hospital staff is a good sign of how patient centered a hospital is and what kind of support it will provide during your recovery from heart surgery and cardiac rehabilitation. A good social worker can provide a treasure trove of helpful information and a good listening ear.

THE 10 BEST QUESTIONS WHEN YOU TOUR A HOSPITAL

Ask yourself this checklist of questions while touring a hospital. Keep your eyes, ears, and nose wide open.

1. How clean is the facility? The patients' rooms?

   Glance into an unoccupied patient room and visitor waiting areas to judge janitorial care.

---

2. Are there any strong odors, particularly of urine or heavy disinfectant?

Trust your nose. Disinfectants can mask serious sanitation problems.

3. How cluttered are the hallways?

A stack of ancient food trays, stinky used linens, or dirty public waiting areas can be a give-away to poor hygiene.

4. How attractive are the patients' rooms?

Look for adequate size and privacy features, like pull curtains or screens, a sunny window, easy television access, and comfortable visitor chairs.

5. How noisy are the hallways? The patients' rooms?

Chronic noise problems plague many hospital patients and can seriously affect your sleep and comfort level.

6. Do the patients' rooms have individual temperature controls? Are the public areas a comfortable temperature?

Like too much noise, too much heat or air conditioning can make you miserable.

7. What are the hospital's policies and accommodations for visitors?

Ideally, visiting hours are reasonable and flexible, and the hospital has facilities (waiting areas, a cafeteria) that are convenient and comfortable.

8. Does the staff speak to the patients — or one another — with disrespect or impatience?

This might be a tip-off that the staff is unhappy, stressed out, and stretched too thin on long shifts.

9. Do nurses and other staff members seem responsive to patients' needs?

Observe if patients' calls for assistance are answered promptly. Check for a bedside call button with easy access.

10. Is the food fresh, attractive, and nutritious?

If needed, ask if arrangements can be made for vegetarian or other special diets. Hospital food often ranks barely above airplane food, but hope for the best with sufficient fresh fruits and vegetables.

The Magic Question

How long are the hallways?

Long hallways together with a nursing staff shortage can seriously delay a nurse's response time to your call for assistance. A poorly designed or disorganized central nurses' station also increases the likelihood of medical errors and lost patient charts.

CONCLUSION

Using the Best Questions in this chapter will help you make a better-informed hospital choice, ensure your safety, and help to speed your recovery from heart surgery or a procedure.

Dr. Larry Hamm concludes, "Hospital stays for heart attacks and surgeries have become greatly compressed to only three to four days nowadays in many cases. This compressed time frame of care increases the importance of asking good questions while you are in the hospital."

THE 10 BEST RESOURCES

Consumers' Checkbook. "Guide to Hospitals." www.checkbook.org. (Subscription required).

HealthGrades.com. "Guidelines for Choosing a High-Quality Hospital." www.healthgrades.com.

Inlander, Charles B., and Ed Weiner. *Take This Book to the Hospital with You: A Consumer Guide to Surviving Your Hospital Stay.* Allentown, PA: People's Medical Society, 1997.

The Joint Commission. "Quality Check Database." www.jointcommission.org. (Accreditation results for specific hospitals.)

Landro, Laura. "The Informed Patient: Hospitals Push to Improve Intensive Care; Effort Seeks to Combat Errors and High Mortality Rates; Giving Beepers to the Family." *Wall Street Journal.* September 25, 2003, p. D1.

Leapfrog Group. "Hospital Ratings." www.leapfroggroup.org/cp.

Sherer, David, and Maryann Karinch. *Dr. David Sherer's Hospital Survival Guide: 100+ Ways to Make Your Hospital Stay Safe and Comfortable.* Washington, DC: Claren Books, 2003.

Smartmoney.com. "10 Things Your Hospital Won't Tell You." www .smartmoney.com/10things/index.cfm?story=october2006.

U.S. Department of Health and Human Services. "Hospital Compare." www.hospitalcompare.hhs.gov.

U.S. News and World Report. "America's Best Hospitals: Heart and Heart Sugery." www.usnews.com/directories/hospitals/index_html/specialty+IHQCARD. (Updated annually.)

CHAPTER 12: THE 10 BEST QUESTIONS
About Cardiac Rehabilitation

Even if you're on the right track, you'll get run over if you
just sit there.

—Will Rogers

Cardiac rehabilitation is a medically supervised outpatient
program to help heart patients recover quickly and improve their physical and mental functioning. Its overall
goals are to slow down or reverse cardiovascular disease, reduce cardiac risk factors, and instill a lifelong love of heart-healthy exercise
and foods.

This rehabilitation is an essential component of recovery care
for heart attack survivors. The current guidelines from the American Heart Association and the American Association of Cardiovascular and Pulmonary Rehabilitation emphasize its importance in
reducing mortality rates, improving quality of life, enhancing psychological recovery, and decreasing the chances for another cardiac
event.

Many heart specialists sing cardiac rehabilitation's praises. A
2004 Mayo Clinic study found that cardiac rehabilitation programs
made a huge difference. Only 5 percent of the patients who went
through rehabilitation died during the three years following their
heart attacks compared to 26 percent of those who did not participate.

Yet participation statistics are dismal. The Mayo Clinic reports that only about half of all heart attack survivors actually
go through cardiac rehabilitation, with even lower rates for
older patients (32 percent after age seventy) and women (only

38 percent of all women). The American Association of Cardio-vascular and Pulmonary Rehabilitation (AACVPR) states that only 10 to 20 percent of patients who need these services receive them.

For heart attack survivors who have never exercised or are obese, it can be a tough lifestyle leap from their couches into a world of gyms, treadmills, and sleek jogging suits. Other survivors are previous fitness enthusiasts but are now too frightened by their cardiac event to resume a regular exercise program.

Sometimes doctors are responsible for low rehab participation rates or are simply not enlightened. Some cardiologists falsely assume that older or obese patients aren't interested. Other doctors just don't give routine referrals.

Let's face it. Doctors don't get reimbursed when you eat your carrots or ride a bicycle. Yet most doctors don't have the time to provide in-depth guidance on the healthy lifestyle changes that are so critical at this point in your life.

Kathy Berra, of Stanford University's Heart Network, says fervently, "Cardiac rehab! Cardiac rehab! Cardiac rehab! It's *so* important. Lower mortality after cardiac rehab has been proven time and time again. If your doctor doesn't refer you to cardiac rehab, ask for it. This should be a joint decision. Cardiac rehabilitation will help you in many, many ways."

Ask your doctor the following 10 Best Questions. Even if your options are limited by your local hospital's offerings, your insurance provider's coverage (most insurance plans and Medicare pay at least partial costs), a rural location, or transportation issues, you owe it to yourself to assess a cardiac rehabilitation program prior to starting it. Ask the program's medical director any questions your doctor can't answer in detail.

THE QUESTION DOCTOR SAYS:

Be your own best advocate. Sometimes you'll need to be persistent in asking your questions.

Keep in mind that some doctors have unspoken biases about patients with your profile (older, woman, nonwhite, overweight, etc.), so be assertive in getting a referral or a solid reason why not. Don't hesitate to ask any other questions that come to mind when you are talking with your doctor or visiting the cardiac rehab center.

>>> THE 10 BEST QUESTIONS
About Cardiac Rehabilitation

1. Am I a good candidate for cardiac rehabilitation? Why or why not?

Many heart attack survivors are surprised to learn that they can begin exercising so soon afterward. Most people are good candidates unless their doctors advise otherwise.

If you think your doctor is stalling or disinterested, ask her what percentage of her cardiac patients she refers to cardiac rehab. Let's hope it's better than 50 percent. Or go find a more enlightened doctor. See chapter 3.

According to the American Association of Cardiovascular and Pulmonary Rehabilitation (AACVPR), the following conditions are appropriate for cardiac rehabilitation. Note that all are covered by Medicare except the last condition. See more at its Web site (www.aacvpr.org/dmtf/cardiacspecific.cfm#arti4):

- Myocardial infarction (heart attack)
- Stable angina
- Heart surgery
- Heart valve replacement or repair
- Percutaneous coronary interventions (PTCA with or without stent)

- Heart transplant or heart/lung transplant
- People at high risk for developing coronary artery disease

2. What will I do in cardiac rehab?

Programs typically consist of several weeks of comprehensive care, including medical evaluation, supervised exercise, discussions on medications and lifestyle changes, smoking cessation, and guidance about resuming your work and regular activities.

You can also expect education and counseling on cholesterol and blood pressure management, weight loss, and healthy diets. Many programs offer emotional and social support, coping with depression sessions, and support groups with other heart attack survivors.

Most programs are offered in phases. For example, phase 1 might consist of education and support that starts during your hospitalization to help you prepare for your life at home after a heart attack. Phase 2 might be a monitored exercise program tailored to fit your individual needs. Phase 3 might be a supervised maintenance program lasting several months. In most cases, a doctor's referral is required for participation.

To learn more about local programs, go to the American Heart Association's Web site: www.americanheart.org/presenter.jhtml ?identifier=10000028. For a sneak preview or as a last-ditch substitute if you can't attend a live session, see the Medline Plus online tutorial at www.nlm.nih.gov/medlineplus/tutorials/cardiacrehabilitation/htm/index.htm.

3. Which cardiac program do you prefer and why? How many referrals have you made to this program? What is the volume (number of patients) in this program?

Assuming you have program choices, a good answer includes a detailed explanation of this program's pros and cons and how it will meet your personal needs. You also want to hear your doctor describe how well and how frequently the program's staff communicates with her about your progress.

Ask, "How often will you receive reports on my progress?" Frequent communication, including exchanging medical records and weekly progress reports, between your doctor and the center is essential. Medicare requires documented interaction throughout the course of the program. It's also an important measure of safety and security from your perspective. Your doctor should not be surprised by this question and should be supportive of your inquiry.

4. Is this program certified by the American Association of Cardiovascular and Pulmonary Rehabilitation (AACVPR)?

All cardiac rehab programs must be operated under the supervision of a physician. However, other than the Medicare guidelines required to treat Medicare patients, no federal license is required. Medicare guidelines are minimal, such as physician supervision and proper emergency equipment.

AACVPR certification is the gold standard for quality in cardiac rehabilitation. Programs must pass a rigorous review every three years of demonstrated outcomes, such as reduced patient angina or fatigue.

To locate your closest AACVPR-certified program, search by state at its Web site (www.aacvpr.org/certification/program_cert_search.cfm). This site also provides the dates a program was certified and provides a contact name and number for each location.

5. How long has this program been in existence?

The longer the better. AACVPR president Dr. Larry Hamm says, "A program that is twenty years old has a lot more experience to draw on than one that's been around for two years. This doesn't mean that the two-year-old program is bad, but it's another piece of data."

6. What kind of volume of patients does this cardiac rehabilitation program have?

The more the better. The logic is that those who do more are better at what they do. A higher-volume program ensures a measure of safety and experience you may not get in a smaller program. Medicare makes decisions on what it will pay for partially based on volume. On balance, remember that smaller or rural communities are likely to have less volume and may still be perfectly acceptable.

7. What are the qualifications of the staff?

According to the AACVPR, staff core competencies should include knowledge and experience with cardiovascular conditions, exercise physiology, diagnostic techniques, metabolic disorders (diabetes, obesity), and the ability to assess cardiovascular capacity. Staffs usually include cardiac nurses, exercise physiologists, physical therapists, and sometimes support group leaders and counselors.

Additional questions to ask about the staff include, "How long have the key staff members worked at this facility?" "What is the ratio of staff to patients?" "How often is there a physician on site?" The gold standard is staff with academic degrees and certifications from the American College of Sports Medicine.

8. Is there a maintenance program? If so, will I be eligible to join it after I complete the standard rehab program?

Many cardiac rehab programs include a phase 3 or phase 4 maintenance program for people who have completed the first two phases and want to continue. Enrolling in a maintenance program is a good idea to help you achieve a permanent commitment to a healthy lifestyle.

Maintenance programs consist of ongoing exercise and education in a supervised environment. Many heart patients prefer to stay with a maintenance program rather than switching to a commercial gym or fitness club.

Being in a supervised program gives you an added measure of safety, and you may be more likely to keep showing up if you have new buddies there who are "just like me"—heart patients, overweight, and reformed couch potatoes. A nominal fee usually applies per session. In most cases, a doctor's referral is required for participation.

9. What are the signs of overexertion while I'm exercising?

Your doctor will likely tell you that you should stop exercising and notify the staff at the cardiac rehabilitation center immediately if you have any of these symptoms:

- Chest pain or discomfort
- A pressure, burning, tightness, or heaviness in your chest
- A racing or skipping heartbeat
- An unusual aching in your arms, shoulders, neck, jaw, or back
- Trouble catching your breath
- Extreme tiredness
- Dizziness, light-headedness, or nausea

Ask your doctor what your target heart rate should be (number of beats per minute). Once you start exercising, ask the person helping you at the cardiac center to show you how to take your pulse on the side of your neck or wrist. Do this frequently while you are exercising to protect yourself. Top athletes monitor their heart rates this way, too.

10. How will I know that I'll be safe from another heart attack during my participation in this program?

Dr. Alfred Bove, president of the American College of Cardiology and a professor emeritus at Temple University Medical Center,

Dr. Larry Hamm, president of the American Association of Cardiovascular and Pulmonary Rehabilitation, says, "We know from previous studies that the most important factor in getting patients to cardiac rehab is the strength of the physicians' referrals. If your doctor says, 'I'll leave it up to you,' that's nothing compared to saying, 'It's *very* important for your full recovery.'"

says, "A cardiac rehab program is an important component of recovery, as it provides a basis for understanding post–heart attack physical capacity and provides the patient with a sense of how much can be done safely."

Asking your doctor this question will help get you over the hump of being afraid or reluctant to start.

❯ The Magic Question

Will you refer me to a cardiac rehab program as quickly as possible? Can I count on your continuing support while I'm in the program?

The probability of effecting meaningful lifestyle changes is never going to be better than it is in the immediate time frame following your heart attack. People are usually highly motivated and supported by their families, including adult children.

You must rely on your doctor's judgment about when you will be strong enough and ready to start rehabilitation. However, some doctors are overly cautious or it just slips their mind.

But timing is crucial. Dr. Larry Hamm says, "Sometimes your opportunity to make heart-healthy lifestyle changes gets lost because it isn't done early enough. If you are six months to one year beyond the acute event, it starts to get repressed in your memory. It's human nature."

Some people get off to a good start but then lose their incentive or support and begin to fall back into bad habits and a sedentary lifestyle. Knowing that your doctor has openly expressed his support will improve your odds of seeing your cardiac rehab graduation day.

CONCLUSION

Cardiac rehabilitation is a total program for heart health. The overall goal of cardiac rehabilitation programs is to help you really make a lifelong commitment to the lifestyle changes that can add years to your life. Think of it as your heart's second chance to keep on pumping.

Dr. Daniel Forman, an assistant professor at the Harvard Medical School and the director of cardiac rehabilitation at the Brigham and Women's Hospital in Boston, says, "Patients often come to cardiac rehab as if it was a bad thing. They say, 'Okay, now I've got to do this.' But I think it's about patient empowerment and should be considered an opportunity, not a punishment."

Dr. Sharonne Hayes, the director of the Mayo Clinic's Women's Heart Clinic, says, "If you are offered cardiac rehab, do it! If you aren't offered rehab, ask for it." Stanford University's Kathy Berra adds, "You must be very, very assertive about this wonderful adventure in your life called cardiac rehab."

Dr. Samuel M. Schwartz, a retired manager at the National Institutes of Health, says it all: "I would highly recommend joining a cardiac rehab program. I had my last heart attack more than twenty-one years ago and here I am. I'm still here!"

THE 10 BEST RESOURCES

American Association of Cardiovascular and Pulmonary Rehabilitation. "Core Components of Cardiac Rehabilitation/Secondary Prevention Programs: 2007 Update." www.aacvpr.org/members/reimbursement/aha _aacvpr_corecomp2007.pdf.

American Association of Cardiovascular and Pulmonary Rehabilitation. "Fast Facts: Referral/Resource Pages for Cardiac Rehabilitation." www .aacvpr.org/dmtf/cardiacspecific.cfm#arti4.

American Association of Cardiovascular and Pulmonary Rehabilitation. "Medical Director Responsibilities for Outpatient Cardiac Rehabilitation /Secondary Prevention Programs." www.aacvpr.org/resources/publica tions/meddirrespon_jcrp2005.pdf.

American Association of Cardiovascular and Pulmonary Rehabilitation. "Program Certification Search." (By state.) www.aacvpr.org/certification/ program_cert_search.cfm.

American Association of Cardiovascular and Pulmonary Rehabilitation. "Resources and Publications." www.aacvpr.org/resources/AACVPRPub .cfm.

American Heart Association. "Cardiac Rehabilitation." www.american heart.org/presenter.jhtml?identifier=4490.

American Heart Association. "What Is Cardiac Rehabilitation?" www .americanheart.org/downloadable/heart/119620120447745%2WhatIs CardiacRehab%209_07.pdf.

Castle Connolly Medical. "Guide to Choosing a Cardiac Rehabilitation Program." www.castleconnolly.com/choiceguides/index.cfm?choice=6.

Mayo Clinic. "Cardiac Rehabilitation: Building a Better Life After Heart Disease." www.mayoclinic.com/health/cardiac-rehabilitation/HB00017.

MetroHealth. "Cardiac Rehabilitation." www.metrohealth.org/body .cfm?id=56&oTopID=56.

CHAPTER 13: THE 10 BEST QUESTIONS

For Choosing Alternative Treatments for Heart Disease

As I see it, every day you do one of two things: build
health or produce disease in yourself.

—Adelle Davis, pioneer nutritionist

The term **alternative medicine** (also called **alternative
treatments** or **alternative therapies**) describes any healing practice that is outside the boundaries of conventional
Western medicine. Common examples include dietary supplements, meditation, naturopathy, herbals, yoga, hypnosis, and chi-
ropractic treatments. Alternative treatments are often used *instead
of* conventional medicine (such as acupuncture to replace pain medications).

In contrast, **complementary medicine** or **complementary
treatments** are used *together with* conventional medicine (such as
therapeutic massage used with a prescription pain medication). The
umbrella term is **complementary and alternative medicine
(CAM)**. The term **integrative medicine** describes a combination
of conventional and CAM therapies.

In reality, all of these terms are often used interchangeably, although some medical professionals prefer clear distinctions. The
definitions are constantly changing as yesterday's CAM treatment
proves safe and effective enough to become today's mainstream
medicine. (Here the terms are used interchangeably, too.)

Alternative therapies for heart health abound because heart disease is so common and potentially deadly. Your choices for alternative treatments are widely diverse, including supplements, herbs,
and vitamins (such as niacin or magnesium); stress-busting tech-

THE QUESTION DOCTOR SAYS:

Check out appealing alternative treatments before your doctor appointment so that you'll be ready to ask your own specific questions on a particular treatment.

niques, like praying or painting; and manipulation and movement, such as tai chi, yoga, and massage.

The good news is about alternative pain relievers that are relatively risk-free (massage, yoga, etc.). The bad news is the lack of standardized federal guidelines for alternative treatments. As a result, a huge market of bogus treatments has sprung up. There are many clever people who make a very good living preying on heart patients by selling them phony products and services.

This chapter has two sets of Best Questions. Ask your doctor the first question set when you are seeking his guidance on alternative treatments. Use the second Best Question list to avoid being scammed by phony heart treatment claims.

>>> THE 10 BEST QUESTIONS
For Choosing Alternative Treatments for Heart Disease

1. Do you think I'm a good candidate for alternative treatments? Why or why not?

Perhaps the most important aspect of this discussion with your doctor is that you are having it at all. Studies show that not many patients who use alternative treatments talk to their doctors about them. Sometimes doctors lack an in-depth knowledge about CAM. Other times, people believe taking supplements or getting a therapeutic massage is a personal decision.

However, you won't know that your supplements are actually

interfering with your regular medications until you have this conversation with your doctor. Dr. Jessica Black, a naturopathic physician in Oregon, advises, "You might be wasting your money on supplements if your body can't absorb these vitamins."

2. Which alternative treatments do you recommend for my physical symptoms? Please explain your rationale.

The CAM choices for pain relief, sleep disturbance, and other typical symptoms are vast because these are also common problems for many people without heart disease. The National Center for Complementary and Alternative Medicine groups CAM treatments into four main categories: (1) whole medical systems, (2) mind–body medicine, (3) biologically based practices, and (4) energy medicine. See its Web site (http://nccam.nih.gov) for details.

An easier classification system divides CAM treatments into two classes: passive and active. A **passive therapy** is one where someone does something to you, such as a massage or acupuncture. An **active therapy** is one where you are the main actor, like attending a yoga class or praying.

Both passive and active treatments can ease your physical symptoms. Be sure you understand your doctor's rationale as well as her specific recommendations for you.

3. Which alternative treatments do you recommend to help me with emotional or psychological issues? Please explain your rationale.

You may need help coping with the psychological or emotional distress that often follows a heart attack or heart disease diagnosis. Alternative treatments aim to balance the whole person—physically, mentally, and emotionally—while standard treatments are doing their job. Some people have stressful lives, depression, or no support system. Again, make sure you understand why your doctor has recommended this therapy and how long you should continue it.

4. What benefits or improvements can I reasonably expect from these treatments?

Your doctor may not know because there is still so much that isn't well understood about how various CAM treatments work. The medical community has only recently become interested in alternative treatments, so there aren't as many evidence-based studies as for more conventional treatments. To see the results on alternative treatment clinical trials for heart disease, go to the Web site www .clinicaltrials.gov, and enter the search terms "heart" and "alternative."

5. Are there any potential side effects or dangers if I use alternative treatments?

There is a wide range of possible side effects across the highly diverse spectrum of alternative treatments. Regardless of the treatment, you want one that's both safe and effective. Ask your doctor if there are treatment standards or guidelines for the recommended alternative treatments you're considering. Discuss your other medical conditions, previous injuries, and current medication regime.

6. In your opinion, do the known benefits outweigh the risks for these treatments?

If the answer is no, explore your doctor's rationale.

7. Are there any alternative treatments that I should totally avoid because they will interfere with my other treatments and recovery?

For example, some herbs can interfere with conventional treatments. Keep in mind the difference between treatments that *add* to conventional treatments and ones that *replace* conventional treatments. Don't substitute unproven herbs for your prescribed blood pressure medicine.

8. Should I let you know before I start an alternative treatment?

This question serves to give you the official stamp of approval on your alternative treatment action plan. Also ask about your doctor's preference for staying informed during the duration of your alternative treatments. You might not want to report every yoga class to your doctor, but give him the option of stating his preferred protocol.

9. What's the best way to find a certified practitioner or learn more about alternative treatments?

Once you have an alternative treatment plan, you'll need a well-qualified practitioner. Rather than holding an MD degree (medical doctor), these practitioners are usually naturopaths, physical therapists, psychologists, or physiatrists (rehabilitation specialists).

Ask a practitioner if he is licensed by a credible institution. Look up this institution on the Internet to make sure it's legitimate. Ask if he belongs to a national association in his field, such as the American Massage Therapy Association (www.amtamassage .org). Ask how many years total experience he has and how many heart patients he's treated in the past.

Interview the practitioner in advance and make sure you feel comfortable. Shop around if needed. Your doctor, support group, or friends can give you referrals.

10. Will this therapy be covered by my insurance?

Alternative treatments run the gamut from free to pricey. Your health insurance provider may not cover the cost or only offer partial coverage. If your doctor or her office staff can't help you with this question, check directly with your insurance company for its fine print before you start any CAM treatments.

❯ The Magic Question

What's the latest reading you've done on CAM or alternative treatments for heart disease?

This question will help you understand your doctor's own personal interest, knowledge, and possible biases about alternative treatments. The reality is that CAM is hot in many medical circles but still ignored by some doctors.

A lot of CAM isn't rocket science but just down-to-earth strategies for a healthier lifestyle and a preventive care mindset. Your doctor will be somewhere along a continuum of involvement with CAM. It makes good sense to understand your doctor's perspective and knowledge base.

THE 10 BEST QUESTIONS TO ASK TO AVOID CAM SCAMS

You are like a dinner bell to con artists promoting bogus heart treatments. These snake oil salespeople prey on heart patients. They know how to take advantage of your pain, emotions, and fears. Even if you think you are too savvy to get scammed, many slick Web sites can fool even the brightest folks.

For example, a so-called miracle cure for atherosclerosis (hardening of the arteries) is **chelation therapy.** The American Heart Association and reputable scientific organizations do *not* endorse this unproven and potentially dangerous therapy. This is just one case where you could waste your money and endanger your health. As Dr. Stephen Barrett of the consumer protection organization Quackwatch, warns, "Don't let desperation cloud your judgment."

The following Best Questions are aimed at Web sites' claims and credentials for providing alternative treatments. You can also easily tailor the questions to use as you review mail advertisements or talk to a salesperson face-to-face.

1. Who's behind this claim or alternative therapy?

Any Web site or company offering medical treatments should offer responsible people's names and their medical credentials. Even if someone sounds impressive, search the Internet for his name and articles in professional medical journals. Run the other way as fast as you can if no one is home at this Web site or company.

2. Are the people offering the alternative therapies also the same people who are selling them?

The funding sources behind a Web site should be clearly explained. Information from a neutral or disinterested third party is usually more reliable than from someone who benefits from product sales.

3. Does this therapy offer a cure, remission, or healing offer?

Alternative therapies like detoxification are not all bad for you or bogus. But some therapies are potentially very dangerous. Avoid Web sites with flowery medical jargon, cure-all claims, multiple ads, and money-back guarantees or free trial supplements.

4. Does the Web site or company have a seal of credibility?

If the Web site or company does not have an approval or accreditation seal, that doesn't automatically make it bogus. But a seal of credibility may provide a measure of quality assurance. Check with Health on the Net Foundation (www.hon.ch) and URAC (www.urac.org) to verify seals.

5. Is this alternative therapy offered as a "miracle" cure for heart disease?

Look out for phrases like "scientific breakthrough," "miraculous cure," "secret ingredient," or "ancient remedy." Don't believe claims that the therapy has "endured for decades or centuries" or that there are many "testimonials" claiming phenomenal success rates.

6. Are any prior studies offered as scientific evidence or are there only anecdotal stories and personal testimonials to back up the claimed benefits of this alternative therapy?

You want specific scientific evidence including measurable results in hard, cold numbers, not that Susie in Georgia liked the taste and felt better afterward.

7. What other documentation is given to support the Web site's or company's claims?

Look for more information, especially in established medical journals, not e-magazines or blogs. Be wary of listings that are old or stopped being updated more than a year ago.

8. Does this alternative therapy or company claim to have exclusive rights to the treatments offered?

Real treatments are widely available and have been used by thousands of heart patients. Fake heart treatments are available from only one doctor, clinic, or Web site. It doesn't make sense that there would be a monopoly on new products or treatments as good as these claim to be.

9. Has any conventional medical organization endorsed this product or treatment?

Endorsements by trusted names in medical science and cardiology are a good sign. In contrast, scammers emphasize that others — usually highly respected doctors or "the establishment" — are trying to suppress the distribution of their products.

10. Is personal information or money requested up front?

Avoid Web sites that won't tell you anything until you've created an account with them and revealed your name, e-mail address, credit card number, or other personal details. Red flags include requests for money up front or perpetual discounts.

The Magic Question

If a medical breakthrough really had occurred in the treatment of heart disease, would the news be announced first in an ad?

The credit for this common-sense Magic Question belongs to the Federal Trade Commission, the federal government's consumer watchdog organization. The con artists' claim of "exclusive rights" is the ultimate tip-off that this is a bogus treatment.

CONCLUSION

According to the National Institutes of Health, about 62 percent of all people with serious illnesses try alternative therapies. The effectiveness of many CAM treatments is still unknown.

Dr. Mimi Guarneri, the medical director of the Scripps Center for Integrative Medicine in La Jolla, California, concludes, "CAM applies to treatment modalities not taught in Western medicine. Our goal is to use global healing traditions that are evidence-based and enhance the practice of conventional medicine."

THE 10 BEST RESOURCES

Barrett, Stephen, and Victor Herbert. "Twenty-Five Ways to Spot Quacks and Vitamin Pushers." www.quackwatch.com/01QuackeryRelatedTopics/spotquack.html.

ClinicalTrials.gov. "All NCCAM Clinical Trials." (Choose "heart failure.") http://nccam.nih.gov/clinicaltrials/alltrials.htm.

Dossey, Larry. *Healing Beyond the Body: Medicine and the Infinite Reach of the Mind.* Boston: Shambhala Publications, 2003.

Guarneri. Mimi. *The Heart Speaks: A Cardiologist Reveals the Secret Language of Healing.* New York: Touchstone, 2007.

Kabat-Zinn, Jon. *Wherever You Go, There You Are: Mindfulness Meditation in Everyday Life,* 10th ed. New York: Hyperion, 2005.

Mayo Clinic. "Complementary and Alternative Medicine." www.mayo clinic.com/health/alternative-medicine/CM99999.

National Center for Complementary and Alternative Medicine. "What Is CAM?" http://nccam.nih.gov/health/whatiscam/.

Oz, Mehmet, and Ron Arias. *Healing from the Heart: A Leading Surgeon Combines Eastern and Western Traditions to Create the Medicine of the Future.* New York: Plume, 1999.

Siegel, Bernie S. *Love, Medicine and Miracles: Lessons Learned About Self-Healing from a Surgeon's Experience with Exceptional Patients.* New York: Harper Paperbacks, 1996.

Weil, Andrew. *Natural Health, Natural Medicine: The Complete Guide to Wellness and Self-Care for Optimum Health,* rev. ed. Boston: Houghton Mifflin, 2004.

PART III

Mending Your Broken Heart with Healthy Lifestyle Changes

A 2006 survey conducted by Mended Hearts, a nationwide heart patient support group, found that most heart attack survivors characterize their heart attack as a life-changing wake-up call. A surprising number of respondents said they feared having another heart attack more than death itself. Yet 40 percent admitted they weren't doing everything possible to avoid one.

That "everything" is making healthy lifestyle changes, such as losing weight, getting more exercise, and stopping tobacco use. Taking care of your heart is now your number one priority. But it's going to take some hard work on your part.

Use the Best Questions in this section to come to grips with whatever unhealthy habits you've slipped into over the years. You didn't develop heart disease overnight, and you won't be able to undo a lifetime of Big Macs, no exercise, and too many cigarettes or drinks overnight, either. Be kind to yourself and try to really be honest with your self-assessment of your stress in chapter 14 and losing weight in chapter 15.

As you transition from a cardiac rehabilitation program, you may be interested in finding a great gym or fitness club (chapter 16) and a top personal fitness trainer (chapter 17) as a strategy to keep up your heart-healthy exercise routines. The last two chapters in this section cover two common health challenges many people face:

quitting smoking (chapter 18) and reducing alcohol consumption (chapter 19).

It's worth it. Even if you've had great doctors, have had an angioplasty or heart surgery, and are on clot-busting drugs, nothing trumps a healthy lifestyle in your battle against heart disease.

CHAPTER 14: THE 10 BEST QUESTIONS

To Tame Your Stress

No one can get inner peace by pouncing on it.
—Harry Emerson Fosdick, American clergyman

There is mounting evidence that stress harms your heart as much as an unhealthy diet and lack of exercise. But because most doctors are extremely busy and are ironically cramming more and more patient appointments into their already crowded calendars, very few have the time to sit and have a long, leisurely physician–patient chat about stress levels. Your doctor may have the best intentions, but realistically she can't do much about the fact that you were laid off from your job last year or that your wife left you last week.

So it's up to you to slow down, take an honest look at what's causing your stress, and consider how much your stress level and emotional state may be affecting your heart's health. The American Stress Institute says that stress management is the one heart disease treatment that many people (and doctors) often overlook as a treatment option.

Reducing stress as a heart disease treatment is probably one of the easiest and safest treatments possible. You can avoid dangerous side effects from drugs, it costs little or nothing, and it has other broader health benefits as well.

Taking the time to slow down and savor the small moments is a life skill that is difficult for most people, but it pays great rewards. Our busy lives keep us moving so fast that we often miss out on the things that are truly important. Each of us has experienced moments of peace, depth, and meaning. But it's tough to make daily relaxation as normal as brushing your teeth.

> **THE QUESTION DOCTOR SAYS:**
>
> Consider seeing a professional counselor or therapist if your stress is out of control or you're having trouble understanding its causes and solutions. To find a reputable therapist, adjust the Best Questions in chapters 3 and 4 and just start asking.

The first step in destressing your life is an honest self-assessment of what's causing your stress. Download all of your free-floating brain and artery-clogging gotta-do's for a few minutes while you ask yourself the following Best Questions.

>>> THE 10 BEST QUESTIONS
To Tame Your Stress

1. When is the last time I felt really relaxed?

Think back. Feel your nerves relax and your throat unclench. What were you doing? Where were you? Why were you relaxed? What relaxes you the most?

Capture your relaxed moments and examine them. What do they have in common? What small piece of this relaxed freedom can you re-create on a daily basis?

This reflection can also be examined from the perspective of the work done by Dr. Herbert Benson, a pioneer in mind-body connections and author of the classic book *The Relaxation Response.* He says, "The Relaxation Response is the biological opposite of the 'fight-or-flight' response. It comes about when you break your train of everyday thoughts by choosing a word to focus on. This word should be repetitive and have meaning, like 'love,' 'peace,' or a prayer."

2. Why am I stressed? What major life changes have I had to deal with within the last year?

From the death of a spouse or a divorce to getting a speeding ticket, stressful events take their toll on our health and well-being. The practical Life Events Questionnaire (also called the Holmes and Rahe Stress Scale) is a list of forty-one stressful life events that can contribute to illness. You can easily take this highly respected and well validated test yourself to assess your risk of stress-induced illness. See http://en.wikipedia.org/wiki/Holmes_and_Rahe_stress_scale.

3. How much is worry or stress affecting my sleep?

Lost sleep robs us of the ability to restore ourselves physically, mentally, and emotionally. Studies done at the University of Chicago found that people who consistently don't get enough sleep have significant metabolic and endocrine changes that mimic the aging process.

Another study found that middle-aged insomniacs have high levels of cortisol, the body's stress hormone. There is also research linking weight gain to sleep deprivation.

Snoring, night sweats, an irritable disposition, daytime sleepiness, difficulty falling asleep at night, sad, angry, or depressed feelings, frequent headaches, and having trouble concentrating are all warning signs that you aren't getting enough quality sleep.

4. Has anyone close to me told me they were worried about my stress level?

Does this sound familiar? Friends and family have pleaded with you, asking for nothing more than a simple phone call. Please, they ask, let me know you're okay.

Or perhaps you've been asked by an old friend, "Are you okay? You don't look so good. Are you still working all that overtime?"

5. If I'm really honest with myself, how much do I think excessive stress contributed to my heart attack?

No one knows the exact correlation yet, but some experts suggest that chronic stress may aggravate the coronary inflammation and blood clots that trigger a heart attack.

A Houston executive and heart attack survivor confessed in a recent business blog, "Although I take pride in being able to spot my employees with too-high stress levels, when my boss called me in last week and said he was worried about my stress level, I was shocked. I seem to know the questions to ask other people about their stress, but I'm clearly missing important clues in my own life."

There are many other contributing factors. For example, a large-scale British study cited in 2008 in the *Harvard Mental Health Letter* found that people who reported toxic relationships with those people closest to them were one-third more likely to have a heart attack or other cardiac event.

6. How much does my job contribute to my stress?

Move over, road rage. Here comes desk rage. And it's getting worse. Anger in the workplace stemming from grumpy coworkers and insulting supervisors, in addition to intense feelings of frustration, fear, and being overwhelmed, is growing.

The American Institute of Stress states that job stress is by far the leading cause of stress for American adults. Eighty percent of workers feel stressed on the job, with nearly half saying they need help. A full 25 percent of American workers view their jobs as the number one stressor in their lives.

Workplace stress consultant Anna Maravelas says, "Be especially careful not to conclude that you're trapped at work. Telling ourselves we have no options causes stress to skyrocket. Instead, be the compassionate witness. If your best friend was describing your work situation to you, what advice would you give him or her?"

Management consultant Sharon Jordan-Evans also offers advice. She says, "As people go into that workplace quandary, 'Should I stay or should I go?' they should first try to find out what's missing and what's wrong in their current job."

7. When I'm stressed, what do I do about it? How well do I recognize stress in myself?

It's important to identify the sources of stress in your life so that you can try to avoid or reduce them. External sources of stress include work pressures, family relationships, and financial worries. There is also self-generated stress in people with type A behavior, which is characterized by a fiercely competitive spirit and unrealistic self-imposed expectations.

Type A behavior can kill. It is a significant risk factor for coronary heart disease and plays a role in elevated cholesterol, hypertension, and smoking.

8. If I wasn't feeling stressed, what would be different?

This question is borrowed from the thinking of **solution-focused brief therapists.** They believe that if people can identify the things they wish they could change in their lives, they are capable of constructing a "preferred future" for themselves. Go to www.sfbta.org.

You can work on developing your own preferred future by asking yourself (or working with a therapist) to construct "what if" questions, like, "What if I woke up tomorrow and a miracle happened that took away all the stress in my life?" "What if I loved my job?" Some people find novel solutions with this innovative approach that examines the gap between the current reality and their ideal state.

9. Do I set standards or expectations for myself that are too high to really achieve?

Many stressed-out people are perfectionists, always striving to get it all right, keep all the balls in the air, and make Superman or Superwoman look like a rookie. Chronic stress can result from a lifelong history of getting straight A's in school, winning key promotions, and expecting your kids to be on the honor roll and be world-class soccer players.

You must consciously break this cycle by seeking stress-reduction techniques, finding more pleasure in smaller sandboxes, and demanding less of yourself and your loved ones. So what if your garden has weeds or your son flunked band class?

10. Who and what can help me the most to reduce the stress in my life?

Stress management gurus advise tackling stress at its root causes. The heart-healthy lifestyle changes you are making (more exercise, healthy diet, etc.) will also tame your stress.

Finding good emotional support can make a huge difference. Consider a support group for heart patients or reconnecting with the people who make you happiest. Find ways to build in more "time-outs" during your everyday life, including quick power naps or meditative moments.

And consider the wisdom of business guru Stephen Covey when he says, "Begin with the end in mind." Charlie Chaplin also got it right when he said, "Nothing is permanent in this wicked world, not even our troubles."

❯ The Magic Question

What is my preferred antidote to stress? How destructive or constructive is it?

Another way of asking this question may be, "What is my favorite poison?" Although some people find smart solutions to stress, like physical activities, favorite hobbies, fun vacations, or playing with their kids, most of us also have destructive behavior patterns that we use as stress reducers.

Cardiac specialist Dr. Daniel Forman of Brigham and Women's Hospital in Boston comments, "Our ways of dealing with stress are often self-destructive, like overeating, smoking, or watching TV." Dr. Herbert Benson adds, "The intensity of a person's fight-or-flight response to stress is determined by that individual's interpretation of its meaning."

Ask yourself whether there is any substance or food that you would have trouble living without. You'll probably immediately consider cigarettes, alcohol, chocolate, fries, or coffee. These addictive stimulants and foods provide short-term energy boosts but can add to your long-term health problems and stress.

A good indication of the impact these substances or foods have on you is what happens when they are withdrawn. For example, many people get headaches when their bodies are deprived of caffeine.

However, such symptoms are usually followed by a feeling of lightness and increased energy as the body is freed from the burden of coping with the toxins created by these substances. Just ask anyone who has successfully quit smoking.

CONCLUSION

Stress is a common medical condition that is largely undiagnosed and untreated in millions of people. Medical research continues to reveal an irrefutable connection between the power of stress and relaxation on our health. Just as stress has a chronic negative effect, regular relaxation has been shown to repair the damage caused by our response to stress.

Live to be one hundred years old. Relax into wellness.

THE 10 BEST RESOURCES

American Institute of Stress. "Topics of Interest." www.stress.org/topic -interest.htm?AIS=9f071b015d36caa499d75130bbaf19b3.

American Psychiatric Association. "Mental Health Resources." www .psych.org/Resources/MentalHealthResources.aspx.

Benson, Herbert. *The Relaxation Response.* New York: HarperCollins, 2000.

Covey, Stephen R. *The 7 Habits of Highly Effective People: Powerful Lessons in Personal Change.* New York: Free Press, 2004.

Kabat-Zinn, Jon. *Wherever You Go, There You Are: Mindfulness Meditation in Everyday Life,* 10th ed. New York: Hyperion, 2005.

Leider, Richard J. *The Power of Purpose: Creating Meaning in Your Life and Work.* San Francisco: Berrett-Koehler, 1997.

Maravelas, Anna. *How to Reduce Workplace Conflict and Stress: How Leaders and Their Employees Can Protect Their Sanity and Productivity from Tension and Turf Wars.* Franklin Lakes: NJ: Career Press, 2005.

Maslach, Christina, and Michael P. Leiter. *The Truth About Burnout: How Organizations Cause Personal Stress and What to Do About It.* Hoboken, NJ: Jossey-Bass, 1997.

University of Massachusetts Medical School. "Stress Reduction Program." www.umassmed.edu/Content.aspx?id=41254.

Wikipedia. "Stress (Biological)." http://en.wikipedia.org/wiki/Stress_%28 medicine%29.

CHAPTER 15: THE 10 BEST QUESTIONS
To Lose Weight and Eat Healthy

I come from a family where gravy is considered a beverage.

—Erma Bombeck

There's a lot of truth to Andy Rooney's observation, "The biggest seller is cookbooks and the second is diet books—how not to eat what you've just learned how to cook."

Many people are confused. For example, top nutritional experts alternatively swear by a dizzying selection of olive oil, no oil, flax-seed oil, butter, margarine, and even lard as best choices. We are bombarded by fad diets, pictures of skinny celebrities and six-pack-ab guys, and tons of tempting sweets everywhere we look. No wonder so many people are overweight or obese.

Your heart attack or heart disease diagnosis may be just the right wake-up call to finally take charge of your weight issues. If so, ask yourself the Best Questions in this chapter. They don't promise a miracle cure, but they can help you understand your own eating behaviors and weaknesses, set realistic long-term goals, and hopefully inspire you to learn more about healthy weight and food choices during your lifetime.

For the Best Questions to ask your *doctor* about weight and diet management, see chapters 7 (risk factors), 8 (women), and 12 (cardiac rehabilitation).

THE QUESTION DOCTOR SAYS:

Why is pie not the answer? It's because the word DESSERTS is STRESSED spelled backward.

>>>THE 10 BEST QUESTIONS
To Lose Weight and Eat Healthy

1. What am I doing to control my portion sizes?

The Muppets' Miss Piggy once said, "Never eat more than you can lift." Portion size has a way of creeping up. We're influenced by a fast-food culture where more food equals better value. It's time to get "unsupersized."

As a registered dietitian in Virginia, Peggy Jensen advises, "People spend a lot of time worrying about *what* they eat but not enough time thinking about *how much* they eat." If you eat half of your normal amounts, you can cut your calories by half without radically changing your favorite foods.

Here are some other time-tested tips. Eat just half a sandwich or half a bowl of ice cream. Chew slowly to let your stomach register it is full. Use smaller salad-sized plates to downsize dinner portions. Buy snacks in smaller bags so that you'll stop sooner. Keep second helpings out of sight. And remember the recommended serving sizes—for example, three ounces of meat is the size of a deck of cards and a cup of potatoes looks like a tennis ball.

2. Am I willing to learn how to read and use the information on food labels?

Besides being a portion-control hawk, the most successful dieters are label fiends. Not knowing how to read the **Nutrition Facts** on labels is a big obstacle in achieving lifetime weight control. A clear explanation is offered by the Food and Drug Administration's Web site at www.cfsan.fda.gov/~dms/foodlab.html.

Also get in the habit of reading the list of ingredients. The list is in descending order by weight. By comparing cereal boxes, for example, you'll see that one brand has more whole wheat and fewer calories than another brand. Choose products with less sodium, corn fructose or corn syrup, saturated fats, and long strings of unappealing chemicals.

As you get more experienced, you'll be able to spot food manufacturers' purposefully misleading statements (reduced-fat crackers with added salt) and confusing bird-sized portions that obscure their real calorie damage.

Cleveland Clinic's preventive medicine consultant, Dr. Caldwell B. Esselstyn advises, "Read the ingredients! And be careful not to get complacent."

3. Would my great-grandmother recognize this food?

Foods are transformed from their original state (like raw vegetables or fresh meat) into marketable food products called **processed foods.** Eating too many highly processed foods is a major cause of weight gain because they often contain refined sugars (think: diabetes epidemic), unhealthy additives, hidden salt and fat, and mystery ingredients (think: hot dogs). The goodness of natural food is usually lost in processing.

The University of Tennessee's nutrition expert Dr. Barbara Clarke comments, "Our food has radically changed. Previously, fast food wasn't so available and grocery stores had limited choices."

Because processed foods are now so commonplace, you might have trouble identifying them. That's why you want to consider your great-grandmother's diet fifty or one hundred years ago. She knew lettuce but not processed vegetable chips and would have recognized frozen cherries but not cherry Kool-Aid.

If you can't channel your great-grandmother, try asking yourself, "Can I pick it, cut it, butcher it, or catch it?" "Would a caveman recognize this food?" Both questions will help you sort out processed and natural food choices.

Dr. Caldwell B. Esselstyn offers a vegetarian version of this Best Question: "Did my food have a face or a mother?" His rules for a simple heart-healthy diet include no meat, fish, chicken, dairy products, salt, eggs, nuts, avocados, oil of any kind (including olive oil), or fruit juice. Eat only whole-grain products and lots of vegetables, fruits, and non-animal proteins.

4. What is my daily allowance for calories, fat grams, fiber grams, salt, and carbohydrates to maintain my weight? To lose weight?

The Recommended Daily Allowance (RDA) describes standard recommendations for a person's intake of essential nutrients to maintain a normal weight and a healthy body. These requirements vary widely based on gender, age, body size, and amount of physical activity.

Many people focus on daily calorie counts, which is a good start but ultimately insufficient for long-term nutritional health. See dietary guidance at this Web site: http://en.wikipedia.org/wiki/Recommended_daily_allowance.

To learn more about how to count your calories for weight loss, see the Calorie Control Council's Web site at www.caloriecontrol.org. If you have only a minimal knowledge about nutrition, ask your doctor or a dietitian for guidance.

5. How frequently can I prepare more of my own food?

If you can cook, you win two big points in the diet war. Preparing at least some meals yourself can be invaluable in weight loss and management because you can control the quality of the ingredients. Dr. Barbara Clarke comments, "It's very important to have cooking skills to manage your diet in a simple, healthful, and controllable way."

Peggy Jensen agrees: "The biggest obstacle is a mindset that I don't have time for this. It's not about preparing foods from scratch but preparing what you eat. When you get into it, you realize it doesn't take more time than the junky stuff or highly-processed convenience food."

6. Who and what can help me achieve my diet and nutrition goals?

Recruit someone more objective about your weight and more knowledgeable about food choices to help you.

Dr. Barbara Clarke says, "If someone is trying to change their diet for medical reasons, they really need to sit down with a registered dietitian and plot out where they are and what can they reasonably change in small steps. We are talking about changing habits that people have had for a long, long time, but we put too much burden on the individual." Likewise, Peggy Jensen suggests, "You can buy shark cartilage on the Web, but a dietitian is going to tell you accurate information and support you."

Experts advise that record keeping is one of the most successful techniques for losing weight. Keep a food diary of everything you eat, its portion size, feelings associated with eating, and calorie count. You'll see patterns emerge that can identify your triggers for overeating. There are many online versions, or try this Web site: http://familydoctor.org/online/famdocen/home/healthy/food/general-nutrition/299.html.

7. Which foods am I willing to give up a few times a week? Which foods would I miss the most?

Without qualifying for full-time martyrdom, consider what bad foods are the easiest to give up, then the second easiest to give up, and so on. Taking your lifestyle changes in small steps will help big time with long-term victory.

Peggy Jensen also suggests asking yourself if you are willing to give up meat a few times a week. This may gradually help you adopt a more plant-based diet.

At the same time, don't forsake your favorite foods forever. Even strict dietitians agree this can be a recipe for a diet disaster. Your intense longing for a favorite food may result in a bingeing session later.

8. What are my smartest choices when I'm dining out?

In advance, check online menus for heart-healthy selections. Ask for a take-out container for oversized restaurant portions or order from the children's menu. Resist upsize offers at fast-food restaurants (the dollar meal deal, etc.), and skip all-you-can-eat buffets.

Instead of choosing the tastiest menu item, retrain yourself to ask, "What is the healthiest thing I can order from this menu?" This wonderful Best Question can rescue you from many diet-sabotaging temptations.

Another consideration is that you may need to be prepared to eat differently from others in a social situation, such as dining at a friend's home. Gently insist that you don't need an overflowing plate or pass on dessert.

9. What is my snack strategy?

Peggy Jensen advises, "When you are hungry, all bets are off. Carry your own healthy snack foods, like nuts or fruit, with you so you won't eat junk food when you are tired or stressed out. When you are hungry, you are mad at the world."

Other smart snack strategies include choosing quality over quantity (a handful of nuts versus a big bag of chips), keeping variety in your snacks (like seasonal fruits, whole-grain crackers, or baby carrots), watching portion sizes, and satisfying cravings with better choices, like yogurt instead of candy or granola bars. Also be careful not to slip up after dinner, a prime time to gain weight because you are probably less active.

10. Is my diet plan one that I can stick with long term?

This diet has to really be your thing, not boring tofu or impossible meals to fix in your already overbooked life. To make your long-term heart-healthy diet and weight loss really work, you first need to internalize this diet—make it work for *you*.

Even if you cook for others, don't cook, or eat out frequently, practicing good nutrition every day is a commitment to yourself. It may take you a few weeks, months, or even years to really get and stay slim.

Work with your doctor or a dietitian to establish short- and long-term goals that are achievable, not just another source of stress for things you haven't done yet. Keep asking yourself Peggy Jensen's question, "What can I eat that is good for me and that I really like?"

❯ The Magic Question

Am I hungry enough to eat an apple?

Many people have been misusing food for so long they are out of touch with their body's true "I'm hungry, feed me" signals. Eating out of habit or to alleviate difficult emotions, such as stress, depression, or fatigue, is very, very common.

One way to get back in touch with your body's true food needs is to choose a food that you like okay, like apples, but don't dream about, like brownies, potato chips, or cheese doodles. Then next time you grab for the cheese doodles, ask yourself this Magic Question. Now, can you put the cheese doodles back?

If you happen to really love apples, find another healthy food for this question. Getting in touch with your pig-out triggers will help you to avoid overindulging in that moment of weakness.

CONCLUSION

Former U.S. surgeon general Dr. Kenneth Moritsugu says, "We doctors can talk until we're blue in the face about the fact that two out of three Americans are now obese or overweight. But only you as an individual have the power to decide whether or not you're going to eat fruits or cookies."

Peggy Jensen concludes by suggesting, "Put a positive spin on your food choices. Rather than grieving for donuts, it's all about finding tasty fruits and vegetables that you really like."

And asking yourself the right questions.

THE 10 BEST RESOURCES

Campbell, T. Colin, and Thomas M. Campbell. *The China Study.* Dallas, TX: Benbella Books, 2006.

Esselstyn, Caldwell B. *Prevent and Reverse Heart Disease: The Revolutionary, Scientifically Proven, Nutrition-Based Cure.* New York: Penguin Group, 2007.

Lillien, Lisa. *Hungry Girl: Recipes and Survival Strategies for Guilt-Free Eating in the Real World.* New York: St. Martin's Press, 2008.

Mayo Clinic. "Food and Nutrition Center." www.mayoclinic.com/health/food-and-nutrition/NU99999.

MedicineNet. "Nutrition Glossary." www.medicinenet.com/script/main/art.asp?articlekey=10366.

National Heart Lung and Blood Institute. "Be Heart Smart! Eat Foods Lower in Saturated Fat and Cholesterol." www.nhlbi.nih.gov/health/public/heart/other/chdblack/smart.pdf.

Oz, Mehmet, and Michael F. Roizen. *You: On a Diet: The Owner's Manual for Waist Management.* New York: Free Press, 2006.

Pollan, Michael. *In Defense of Food: An Eater's Manifesto.* New York: Penguin Press, 2008.

Schlosser, Eric. *Fast Food Nation.* New York: Harper Perennial, 2005.

Zinczenko, David, and Matt Goulding. *Eat This Not That: Thousands of Simple Food Swaps That Can Save You 10, 20, 30 Pounds—or More!* Emmaus, PA: Rodale, 2007.

CHAPTER 16: THE 10 BEST QUESTIONS
To Find a Great Gym or Fitness Club

You have to stay in shape. My grandmother, she started
walking five miles a day when she was sixty. She's ninety-
seven today and we don't know where the hell she is.
> —Ellen DeGeneres

Belonging to a gym or fitness club (the terms are used interchangeably here) can be a great motivator if you choose the
right one and get prior approval from your doctor. Implement-
ing a regular exercise routine is a very positive step in your battle against
heart disease. Having a comfortable place to go that supports your fitness goals will help you keep on track. And you might even have fun.

If you are in a cardiac rehabilitation program, ask your doctor
about continuing with its long-term maintenance program. Dr. Daniel Forman, an assistant professor at Harvard Medical School and director of cardiac rehabilitation at the Bingham and Womens' Hospital
in Boston, says, "People who start exercising on their own in a ran-
dom way are usually the ones who find less value in their exercise
routines and end up stopping. Supervised people do much better."

If you want to exercise independently or with a personal trainer
at a fitness club, ask the membership director or other representative
these following Best Questions while you are touring the facility.

>>> THE 10 BEST QUESTIONS
To Find a Great Gym or Fitness Club

1. What activities and support services are available here?
This is ultimately the deal-breaker question. If you want water aerobic classes but there's no pool in this fitness club, you'll have to

> **THE QUESTION DOCTOR SAYS:**
>
> Try to tour several local fitness centers before you make your final decision. Make extra copies of these Best Questions so that you can ask questions at each facility and compare answers later.

look elsewhere. You may want yoga classes, tai chi, massages, or walking programs, but this club only offers kickboxing and step aerobics.

Follow-up questions include, "May I see a class schedule?" "What services do you have for cardiac patients or seniors?"

Also check to see if any of this club's advertised activities have additional charges or hidden fees. Some popular classes like yoga may cost extra.

2. Where is the gym located?

A key consideration in choosing a fitness club is its location. The ideal travel time is fifteen minutes or less. Make sure that parking won't send you off to the Dairy Queen in frustration.

Bill Sonnemaker, MS, an international award-winning master personal trainer and the CEO of Catalyst Fitness in Atlanta, advises, "The closer and easier it is to get to, the less likely you'll be to come up with an excuse for not going regularly. Make sure your drive is as short as possible so you can't use the excuse, 'There's not enough time to exercise.'"

3. When is the gym open?

Check the hours to make sure they are easy to fit into your schedule. Decide for yourself what time of day you are most likely to use the facility.

Come back unannounced on another day during your preferred

time to see how crowded the gym is and to check out en route traffic conditions.

4. Are the staff members degreed and certified?

Dr. Larry Hamm, a cardiac rehabilitation specialist at The George Washington University, warns, "Most of the fitness clubs, not all, but most clubs hire personal trainers who are only minimally qualified without requiring any kind of college degree or a degree in exercise science or exercise physiology."

One quality check is to ask if this facility belongs to a professional fitness association, such as IDEA (www.ideafit.com) or IHRSA (www.ihrsa.org). Make sure the staff's personal certifications are from an accredited organization discussed in chapter 17.

5. How old is the equipment?

Do you see any equipment with "Out of Service" signs? Ask how often the equipment is cleaned for health and safety purposes.

6. How well designed and maintained is this facility?

The group exercise floor should be designed to provide shock absorption. Look for instructions conveniently posted for each piece of equipment. Are there enough machines so that you won't have to wait to use them? Is there enough space between machines so that you don't bump into other people? Is the pool area clean and easily accessible?

Are there gathering areas where people can sit and socialize? Is the facility bright and cheerful and the noise level tolerable?

7. How clean and comfortable is the locker room?

Check out the locker room area for cleanliness and roominess, a comfortable temperature, and good lighting. Are there any dangerous areas—for example, loose tiles or carpet edges—that could cause a fall? Are towels, soap, and shampoo provided or can you obtain them for an extra charge? Is there a shower stall with wheelchair accessibility?

8. Has anyone ever been hurt here? What emergency procedures do you have in place? Do you have an automated external defibrillator on the premises?

You may not get an honest answer, but ask anyway. Also ask if this facility carries liability insurance in case you get injured.

The entire staff should have completed cardiopulmonary resuscitation (CPR) training at bare minimum. Anyone trained to operate an automated external defibrillator must also be trained in CPR, since early CPR is a critical step in resuscitation to help reestablish the circulation of blood and oxygen.

Ask the staff what they would do if someone had a heart attack on their premises. If they don't say "call 911 immediately," don't go there.

9. What are the terms of the contract?

Don't get roped into an extended contract, especially if you aren't sure how committed you are at this point. There shouldn't be any pressure to sign anything, especially a long-term agreement. Ask if you can try the club for a couple of weeks or start with a month-to-month membership.

Other good follow-up questions include, "Are there any services, classes, or amenities that cost extra?" "Will the club offer a trial membership or waive the initiation fee?" "What is your cancellation policy (and any penalties)?"

Price depends on geographic location and how nice the facility is. Decide on your price range ahead of time. Most facilities charge between $30 and $50 or more per month.

Assess later if this facility seemed more service oriented or sales oriented. Bill Sonnemaker, MS, explains, "The staff should encourage you to *use* the facility, not just belong."

10. What is the atmosphere and "personality" of this fitness club?

Paige Waehner, a certified personal trainer and author in Chicago, says, "You want to feel comfortable in your workout environment. If you walk in and the music is too loud, the floor is very crowded, or you feel overwhelmed by all the machines and gadgets, you'll be less likely to show up for your workouts."

Look around and decide if the clients are people who you can relate to. Do they look happy or stressed out? Socializing at a fitness club will keep you coming back because you develop workout buddy friendships.

How many people are working with personal trainers? Do the trainers look bored or are they actively engaged? Sonnemaker says, "The bottom line here is when you walk into a club you should feel comfortable, as if you belong there."

〉 The Magic Question

Does this facility belong to the Medical Fitness Association?

Perhaps you've never heard of medical fitness centers because there's not one on every street corner. Dr. Cary Wing, executive director of the Medical Fitness Association, explains, "By definition, a medical fitness center must have either a medical director or a physician advisory board that oversees the program, although the supervision may not be full-time."

Most medical fitness centers are affiliated with a hospital, health care system, or physicians' practices. They differ from regular gyms because the staffers are exercise physiologists, physical therapists, or athletic trainers with nationally recognized certification and experience in helping people transition from cardiac rehabilitation programs.

This is good news and an extra measure of safety for you as a recovering heart attack or heart disease patient. These facilities are more likely to do an initial full health risk assessment, taking your cardiac history and other medical conditions into consideration; require higher standards of qualifications and performance from their staff; and know about heart medications and exercise limitations.

There are currently about 950 medical fitness centers in the United States, with the numbers growing to meet the health needs of an aging population. See their Web site at www.medicalfitness .org.

CONCLUSION

Asking the right questions before joining a gym can save you a ton of money and ensure your health and safety are in good hands. Once you get your doctor's approval for exercising, look for a fitness center that matches your needs and style. Dr. Cary Wing advises, "There's an intimidation factor in a fitness center for many people."

No matter how fancy a health club is, your ultimate Best Question is, "Will I keep coming back?" Paige Waehner concludes, "Ask yourself if this is a place you can see yourself going to on a regular basis." All the latest equipment, the nicest showers, or the world's best personal trainers won't do you a bit of good if you don't actually use the facility.

THE 10 BEST RESOURCES

AARP. "Choosing a Health & Fitness Club." www.aarpfitness.com/articles.aspx?articleID=1005.

American College of Sports Medicine. "Physical Activity and Public Health in Older Adults: Recommendations." www.acsm.org/AM/Text

Template.cfm?Section=Home_Page&Template=/CM/ContentDisplay
.cfm&ContentID=7789.

American Council on Exercise. "Before You Start an Exercise Program."
www.acefitness.org/fitfacts/fitfacts_display.aspx?itemid=94.

American Council on Exercise. "Exercising with Heart Disease." www
.acefitness.org/fitfacts/fitfacts_display.aspx?itemid=34.

American Council on Exercise. "Fit Facts: Cardiovascular Exercise." www
.acefitness.org/fitfacts/default.aspx#Choosing%20Fitness%20Trainers%20
and%20Instructors.

American Council on Exercise. "How to Choose a Health Club." www
.acefitness.org/fitfacts/fitfacts_display.aspx?itemid=111.

International Council on Active Aging. "How to Select an Age-Friendly
Fitness Facility." www.icaa.cc/facilitylocator/ICAA%20Facility%20Test
.pdf.

Mayo Clinic. "Fitness." www.mayoclinic.com/health/fitness/SM99999.

Medical Fitness Association. *The Medical Fitness Model: Facility Standards
and Guidelines.* Richmond, VA, 2008.

Sonnemaker, Bill. "How Fitness Aids in Rehabilitation." www.fitness
catalyst.com/Current-Articles.html.

CHAPTER 17: THE 10 BEST QUESTIONS

To Hire a Top Personal Trainer

> Whether you think you can or think you can't, you're
> right.
>
> —Henry Ford

L ike any other profession, personal fitness training attracts its
share of losers. In fact, trainers' missing credentials are often
ignored, especially if they look like bodybuilding rock stars.
There are many mediocre people in this field who lack depth in education and experience.

Having a personal trainer you trust can make all the difference
if you are transitioning from a cardiac rehabilitation program with
its highly structured, customized exercises to the real world of commercial gyms and fitness clubs. Besides, Oprah and many other rich
and famous people have their own personal trainers, so why not
you? But how do you find a great trainer?

If your cardiac rehabilitation program offers you a maintenance
program for a reasonable fee, ask your doctor about staying with it
for your long-term physical activity needs. If not, these Best Questions are for you when you interview potential personal trainers before signing a contract.

Bill Sonnemaker, MS, an internationally award-winning master
personal trainer and the CEO of Catalyst Fitness in Atlanta, and
Paige Waehner, an experienced certified personal trainer and author
in Chicago, provided substantial assistance in developing the following Best Questions.

>>>THE 10 BEST QUESTIONS
To Hire a Top Personal Trainer

1. Are you certified by an accredited organization? If so, which one?

"Over 95 percent of people practicing as personal trainers should not be doing so, because they are not certified by an accredited and medically recognized organization," according to Bill Sonnemaker. There are over three hundred personal trainer certification programs, but only four are accredited by third parties and recognized by the medical community.

Look for a certification from one of these four organizations: the National Academy of Sports Medicine (NASM), the American Council on Exercise (ACE), the National Strength and Conditioning Association (NSCA), and the American College of Sports Medicine (ACSM).

Bill Sonnemaker adds that the gold standard for someone recovering from a heart attack is the American College of Sports Medicine, especially with ACSM's certification designation of "health and fitness instructor" or "exercise specialist." ACSM was founded on cardiac rehab and aerobic exercise, but it is weaker on resistance training and flexibility exercises. In Sonnemaker's opinion, the National Academy of Sports Medicine offers the best overall well-rounded certification programs for trainers and excels at designing its exercise programs.

2. How long have you been a personal trainer?

Look for someone with enough experience to be able to anticipate your needs and safety issues, keep you motivated, and who feels comfortable talking to your doctor. Avoid the burned-out, bored, or cynical types who would rather chit-chat or sit and watch while you sweat it out on a treadmill. Experience is no guarantee, but it helps.

3. What specific experience and education do you have for working with cardiac patients?

The more details she gives you, the better. Insist on actual time as a personal trainer, not personal time developing her own personal workout routines.

Ask about her specific training for health-challenged clients, her plans for keeping you safe, and numbers and dates (how long together and how long ago) for her past cardiac patients. Ideally, your trainer also has some college education, preferably a bachelor's degree in exercise physiology.

4. When is the last time you completed a continuing education course? Did you take this class online or with a live instructor?

The best fitness instructors complete a minimum of twenty training hours every two years. This is equivalent to attending a two-and-one-half day course or three-day conference.

"Be leery of trainers who only do correspondence courses," says Bill Sonnemaker. "True professionals spend the money to attend a conference so they can learn from others and from the best people in the industry."

5. How do you plan to personalize my training program?

Paige Waehner advises, "The best exercise plan involves activities that are accessible and enjoyable. If you enjoy what you're doing, you're much more likely to do it on a regular basis while having fun."

Find out what kind of exercises you'll be doing. Your trainer may need more time to figure out a detailed exercise plan, but the most important thing to listen for is a tailored, individualized plan for you, not just a cookie-cutter exercise solution.

6. How will you help me to meet my fitness goals?

A trainer needs to be knowledgeable and wise enough to find the right balance between keeping you safe and pushing your heart toward a healthy workout. Sonnemaker advises, "The doctor may have released you for exercise, but sometimes the trainer is too cautious. It's always better to err on the side of caution, but at the same time you want some stress (exercise intensity) on your system, which needs to be determined by your physician."

Another quality indicator is how well organized a trainer is. Look for someone who will keep notes on your progress and can temporarily transfer your records to another trainer if he is out sick.

7. What is your follow-up strategy?

The best trainers anticipate the day you'll leave them to exercise independently on your own. To accomplish this, they typically give "homework"—exercises to do in between your gym sessions together.

Ask if this trainer has printed handouts on exercises and will give you copies so that you can do the exercises correctly later. It's one thing to watch your trainer demonstrate an exercise but another thing to try to repeat it by yourself. This strategy will help you to prevent injuries or overexert yourself.

8. Do you have professional liability insurance?

This matters to you because it shows a higher level of professionalism and protects you in case you get hurt and it's the trainer's fault. If the trainer doesn't have liability insurance and you've got medical bills as a result of something this trainer did or didn't do, you're out of luck.

9. What are your hourly rates? Do you have any discounts or other offers? Can I try a sample session for free?

Rates vary according to geographic location and a trainer's qualifications, ranging between $50 and $100 or more per hour. Keep in mind that the cheapest trainer in town may not be able to help you reach your goals.

Some trainers offer free or reduced prices for a get-acquainted or trial session. You won't know until you ask!

10. Could you please give me the names and contact details for three of your clients who I can check with?

Ask for referrals to other cardiac patients or people similar to you, not teenagers or professional athletes. Then really follow through on your calls. These referrals can provide a wealth of information.

Ask: "Why did you like this trainer?" "Was there ever a time that you questioned his judgment about your safety or well-being?" "Would you send your friends or family to this trainer?"

❯ The Magic Question

How do you plan to stay in communication with my doctor? How often?

Bill Sonnemaker says, "It's important that the trainer has immediate interaction with the physician and with any of the therapists in cardiac rehab. Doctors are going to be more specific when they are writing things down than over the phone, because they realize their own liability. A really savvy trainer will have either an e-mail or fax communications going on with the doctor that includes telling the

THE QUESTION DOCTOR SAYS:

In addition to reflecting how this trainer reacted to your questions, also consider how many questions he asked you. Did he ask these questions with genuine interest and listen intently or did this trainer just seem to be going through the motions?

Best Question 5 should have prompted this person to ask you for details on your fitness goals. This little insight might say a lot about how likely this trainer is to go the extra mile for you.

doctor about the training program and what types of exercises we are proposing."

Paige Waehner adds, "You want to make sure your trainer is willing to reach out and accept help and guidance from other resources including your doctor or physical therapist."

CONCLUSION

If you are coming out of cardiac rehab, a personal trainer can keep you motivated and organized in your exercise goals, especially if you are a former couch potato. However, you don't want a muscle-bound beach bum who's just masquerading as a personal trainer.

Keep in mind that your timing is critical. If you've just been released from your cardiac rehab program, you don't want to lose all those positive gains you've made and slide back into a sedentary lifestyle. Working with a credentialed, experienced trainer can help you to internalize a lifelong commitment to getting more physical activity.

Verify your exercise goals with your doctor before you start with any independent program or trainer. And keep checking to make sure your personal trainer and doctor are still communicating regularly about your progress.

THE 10 BEST RESOURCES

American College of Sports Medicine. "Selecting and Effectively Using a Personal Trainer." www.acsm.org/AM/Template.cfm?Section=Brochures 2&Template=/CM/ContentDisplay.cfm&ContentID=8103.

American Council on Exercise. "Fit Facts™: Choosing Fitness Trainers and Instructors." www.acefitness.org/fitfacts/default.aspx#Choosing%20 Fitness%20Trainers%20and%20Instructors.

American Council on Exercise. "How to Choose an Online Personal Trainer." www.acefitness.org/fitfacts/fitfacts_display.aspx?itemid-116.

American Council on Exercise. "How to Choose the Right Personal Trainer." www.acefitness.org/fitfacts/fitfacts_display.aspx?itemid=19.

Aquatic Exercise Association. "H20 Personal Training." www.aeawave .com/PublicPages/Home/tabid/54/ctl/DetailView/mid/457/itemid/110/ Default.aspx.

Catalyst Fitness. "Choosing a Personal Trainer." www.fitnesscatalyst.com/ Choosing-a-Personal-Trainer.html.

International Council on Active Aging. "How to Choose an Age-Friendly Personal Trainer." www.icaa.cc/facilitylocator/icaapftguide.pdf.

National Strength and Conditioning Association. "Find a Trainer." www .nsca-lift.org.

Waehner, Paige. About.com. "Choosing a Personal Trainer." http:// exercise.about.com/cs/forprofessionals/a/choosetrainer.htm.

Waehner, Paige. About.com. "Why a Trainer May be Right for You." http://exercise.about.com/cs/forprofessionals/a/choosetrainer.htm.

CHAPTER 18: THE 10 BEST QUESTIONS

To Break Nicotine's Grip

Failure should not be our undertaker, but our teacher.

—Denis Waitley, American speaker and author

Yes, you can quit smoking—for good. What's going to make the crucial difference this time is your experience of surviving a heart attack or getting a diagnosis of severe heart disease. Thousands of ex-smokers who have already quit did so because they realized that their heart event or diagnosis was the most important wake-up call of their lives.

Getting out of Marlboro country forever is the single best thing you can do for your heart health. Second heart attacks are twice as common for cardiac patients who continue to smoke. Period.

Smoking isn't a habit; it's an addiction. Pure willpower as the sole weapon for battling this addiction usually isn't enough for most people. Quitting tobacco can't be compared to breaking a potato chip or chocolate habit. It's closer to quitting heroin.

If you've had a hard time trying to quit—and staying quit— talk to your doctor for advice. Get help from your cardiac rehabilitation program. Join a support group. There are many Web sites and books available, including the ones listed at the end of this chapter and the end of this book.

It will also help you if you try—really, really try—to *honestly* understand yourself and why you smoke or use tobacco. Asking yourself the following Best Questions is a good start on your journey to a smoke-free and longer life. Ask your doctor the second set of Best Questions to get her guidance.

THE QUESTION DOCTOR SAYS:

Some people come to see their cigarettes as a friend they can count on for comfort and companionship. Quitting can be like losing that friend. No wonder this is so tough.

Women who smoke have heart attacks more than a dozen years earlier than women who don't smoke, according to a 2008 Norwegian study. Your "friend" is killing you.

>>>THE 10 BEST QUESTIONS
To Break Nicotine's Grip

1. Why do I want to quit smoking?

The best answer is "for me." If you aren't doing it for you but for someone or something else in your life, experts agree it's not going to work.

Dr. Edwin B. Fisher, professor, author, and a world-renowned expert on smoking behavior, advises, "The more people can personalize the reasons they want to quit, the more they will be able to stay off cigarettes. You need to make this motivation very concrete. For example, you might say to yourself, 'Although I've had a heart attack, I still want to see my grandchildren graduate from high school.'"

2. What problems, triggers, and obstacles am I likely to encounter?

Anticipating and planning for problems ahead of time is one of the best things you can do for yourself. How will you deal with your urges? What situations trigger a cigarette craving? What times of the day are you most vulnerable?

You must get rid of all temptations. Trash your cigarette stash, ashtrays, lighters, and any other reminders. To quit smoking, you have to get rid of the things that make it possible. If you live with a smoker, ask him or her to quit with you or not smoke in front of you.

3. Do I smoke in order to relax or feel better? If so, what can I use as a substitute for stress relief?

All sorts of emotions become linked with smoking. The most common form of psychological dependency is to use cigarettes to cope with stress, anxiety, or depression. Other people love to smoke when they are having fun, working, or feeling creative. "Nicotine is a great drug to elevate mood and help you to wake up, but the delivery method is lethal," says Dr. Edwin B. Fisher.

People think cigarettes help them relax. Wrong. What cigarettes actually do is calm your nicotine cravings for the next cigarette.

You can reduce your stress by taking a hot bath, exercising, or reading a book. Try not to use food as a substitute stress reliever. Many people do, which partially explains why weight gain is so common after quitting.

4. What lessons have I learned from my past attempts to quit smoking?

The American Lung Association's national program manager for smoking cessation, Bill Blatt, says, "Realizing that you aren't a bad person because you haven't been able to quit is huge. A lot of smokers look back and think about how many times they tried to quit and that it never worked before."

Okay, so instead of beating yourself up about failed past attempts, what did you do *right*? And what did you learn about yourself that you can do again? Try to remember specifically what you did during the times that you successfully resisted urges to smoke.

Bill Blatt suggests you think of your past attempts as your "practice quits," not as failures.

5. Which of my daily activities are most strongly associated with having a cigarette? How can I break the association between these activities and smoking?

There are many links between you and your cigarettes that you may not even realize. You might have started out smoking during coffee breaks with office friends, but now you always want a cigarette anytime you have coffee.

Maybe it's the first cigarette in the morning or the smoke after dinner that will be the hardest to give up. Other common activities are talking on the telephone, watching television, driving, socializing, and after eating. Dr. Edwin B. Fisher says, "People need to identify the situations that are really going to be tempting for them."

Think about it. When do you automatically reach for a cigarette? Plan on alternative activities, like skipping coffee breaks, watching television in a different chair, or anything else that will help you break these deep-seated habits.

6. When is my Quit Day? How can I personalize this day to really mean something to me?

About one-third of heart attack survivors quit smoking while they are still in the hospital after their surgery. Being hospitalized forces quitting.

If you haven't already quit and want to try to quit within the next month, Dr. Edwin B. Fisher advises, "The more specific you can make your Quit Day in terms of place, time, and activity, the better. Someone might want to quit on Monday because their workplace has such strict restrictions on smoking that it makes it easier for them than quitting on a weekend." Or choose a birthday, anniversary, or another special date.

Be smart. Plan your own Quit Day in specific detail in advance so that you'll make a strong personal commitment to be a winner.

7. Do I want to take medication to help me quit smoking?

Medicines or products that help you get over a physical addiction to nicotine are called **nicotine replacement therapies (NRT)**. These medications or products ease nicotine withdrawal and cravings. They are generally considered to be useful and safe in most people with heart disease when used as a part of a comprehensive smoking cessation program. However, consult with your doctor first to be sure. Your doctor may also offer you a prescription antidepressant, such as bupropion (Zyban) or varenicline (Chantix).

Different people do better with different methods. You can choose from one of these types:

- Nicotine patch
- Nicotine gum
- Nicotine inhaler
- Nicotine lozenge
- Nicotine nasal spray

The gum and patches are available at your local pharmacy. Ask your doctor for a prescription for one of the other medications.

The American Heart Association reports that consistent use of one of these NRT products doubles a person's chances of quitting smoking.

8. Who will be my best advocates to help me quit smoking? Who will be least supportive?

Twenty-six percent of ex-smokers in a 2007 poll cited by *USA Today* said their primary factor in successfully quitting smoking was the support they received from their family and friends. Gather your most supportive allies around you and let them know your plans to quit.

Which of your friends (like bar or poker buddies) are most likely to be a bad influence while you are trying to quit? Try to avoid these people (and situations), at least for a while.

Support groups can be very useful. See chapter 23. Get help from the National Network of Tobacco Cessation Quitlines (www.smoke free.gov/expert.html) or call toll free 1-800-QUIT NOW. There are thousands of local quit chapters and telephone counselors to help you.

9. How will I cope with the possibility of gaining weight?

Rats on nicotine eat less, especially sweets. The same is true for people, which means you are likely to face weight gain. Consider this in advance so that you'll be ready to deal with it. Get all tempting foods out of your home ahead of time.

Statistically, most people gain ten pounds or less. Talk to your doctor for advice and ask him the Best Questions below.

10. How can I make living without tobacco my lifelong goal?

This question may take you back to the first Best Question about your motivation to quit smoking. Now you are looking at your long-term goal to live a full life without cigarettes.

According to the U.S. Surgeon General's Office, ten years after quitting, your risk of lung cancer is about one-third to one-half that of continuing smokers. Fifteen years after quitting, your risk of heart disease is that of a nonsmoker's. That's a wonderful goal to strive for.

❯ The Magic Question

What else can I do with my hands when I'm trying to quit smoking?

Holding a cigarette, tapping out the ashes, and drawing your cigarette to your face are deeply ingrained pleasurable habits you are only slightly aware of until you try to quit smoking.

Ask almost anyone who has tried to quit smoking and they'll tell you they miss the comfortable feelings associated with touching and handling cigarettes. In fact, many smokers say they've gone back to smoking because, "I had nothing to do with my hands."

Pick up a pen or pencil, doodle, play with a coin or a ring, or take up a hobby that keeps your hands busy—anything to break the hand-mouth-cigarette association.

THE 10 BEST QUESTIONS TO ASK YOUR DOCTOR ABOUT QUITTING SMOKING

Ask your doctor these questions to get medical advice and to boost your motivation to quit smoking.

1. What are my health risks if I don't quit smoking?

You probably already know the evils of tobacco, but there's nothing like hearing it again from your cardiologist to make it really sink in.

2. Can I use a nicotine replacement therapy?

Ask which type your doctor recommends and for a prescription, if needed.

3. After I quit, when will the urges stop? What can I do about cravings?

Try to get some practical tips from your doctor on these important questions.

4. How can I keep from gaining weight?

Many people gain some weight and find this so discouraging that they start smoking again. Get practical advice on avoiding this problem.

5. If I have to choose between quitting smoking and gaining weight, which is more important?

There's a strong chance your doctor will tell you to lose the cigarettes, but hearing it from him may strengthen your resolve.

6. How much weight can I afford to gain if I quit smoking?

Hearing a number will help you clarify and set realistic goals.

7. What if I slip and go back to smoking?

Your doctor may be able to prescribe a different nicotine replacement therapy or offer medical advice.

8. Should my partner and I quit together?

This answer partially needs to come from you, but see what your doctor says as well.

9. What are the effects of secondhand smoke on my children, family, and friends?

Sometimes hearing from a doctor how your smoking hurts the ones you love can be another powerful incentive to quit.

10. Do you have someone on your staff I can talk with for counseling and questions?

Many doctors use a physician assistant or nurse practitioner. Ask for this person's name and telephone number.

The Magic Question

How soon after I quit will I experience health improvements?

You'll enjoy hearing from your doctor that twenty minutes after quitting your heart rate and blood pressure drops, twelve hours after quitting the carbon monoxide level in your blood returns to normal, and one year after quitting the excess risk of coronary heart disease is half that of a smoker's, according to the American Cancer Society.

CONCLUSION

Nicotine reaches the brain in just seven seconds after each drag. A pack-a-day smoker takes seventy thousand "hits" a year. This is a very powerful drug. A major study in Norway found that people who smoke only one to four cigarettes per day are still significantly increasing their risk of death from heart disease.

The American Lung Association's Bill Blatt says, "It took a while for most people to learn how to smoke. It's going to take a while to learn how to quit. But I believe that every smoker can quit. It might not be easy, but you can quit."

A known enemy is more easily overcome. After your heart attack, there's no shred of doubt that tobacco is your enemy. There are forty-six million Americans who are ex-smokers with success stories. It's time to join them or ask yourself, "Why not?"

THE 10 BEST RESOURCES

American Cancer Society. "Guide to Quitting Smoking." www.cancer.org /docroot/PED/content/PED_10_13X_Guide_for_Quitting_Smoking. asp?sitearea=PED.

American Heart Association. "Medicines to Help You Quit Smoking." www.americanheart.org/presenter.jhtml?identifier=3048078.

American Heart Association. "No-Smoking Confidence Assessment and Tips." www.americanheart.org/downloadable/heart/1184610986257DO WNLOADASSESSMENT2%20071607%20FINAL.pdf.

American Lung Association. "Local Chapters." www.lungusa.org/site /apps/kb/zip/zip.asp?c=dvLUK9O0E&b=37083.

American Lung Association. "Smoking Cessation Support." www.lungusa.org /site/c.dvLUK9O0E/b.22931/k.8550/Smoking_Cessation_Support.htm.

HealthGrades. "Smoking and Risk of Heart Attack Quiz." www.health grades.com/health-management-tools-directory/smoking-and-risk-of-heart-attack-quiz.htm.

National Network of Tobacco Cessation Quitlines. Toll-free hotline: 1-800-QUIT NOW (1-800-784-8669). www.naquitline.org.

Nicotine Anonymous. "Welcome." www.nicotine-anonymous.org.

Peele, Stanton. *7 Tools to Beat Addiction.* New York: Three Rivers Press, 2004.

SmokeFree.gov. "Clearing the Air: Quit Smoking." www.smokefree.gov/ pubs/clearing_the_air.pdf.

CHAPTER 19: THE 10 BEST QUESTIONS

To Assess Your Drinking Habits

When I read about the evils of drinking, I gave up reading.

—Henny Youngman, American comedian

Sometimes it's hard to know the right thing to do. Research studies have indicated that moderate alcohol consumption might actually be good for you. Moderate drinkers are less likely to suffer heart attacks than abstainers or heavy drinkers and are more likely to enjoy greater longevity.

For example, Harvard researchers looked at thousands of physicians with similar lifestyles and health conditions. They found that people who had the same lifestyle and drank alcohol had better cardiac health. Italians, Greeks, and other native Mediterranean people whose "Mediterranean diet" has won widespread heart-healthy acclaim typically drink alcohol with their meals.

The best-known positive effects of alcohol on the heart are its anticlotting properties and a small increase in HDL (good) cholesterol, although regular exercise can achieve the same effects. Recent research has found that if you both exercise and drink in moderation, the cumulative effects are even better than doing just one of these without the other. But there continues to be medical controversy over whether moderate consumption of beer, wine, or distilled spirits decreases the risk of heart disease. Studies suggest that they are effective, with each having an equal advantage.

Dr. David J. Hanson, an internationally recognized alcohol consultant and professor in New York, says, "Red wine is a controversial subject. Basically, the research does not consistently demonstrate any superiority of wine over beer or other spirits. There really isn't any good evidence that red wine has any special protective properties. The primary benefit seems to be in the alcohol itself."

The American Heart Association recommends that if you drink alcohol, you should do so in moderation. The U.S. Department of Health and Human Services defines moderate drinking as no more than one drink a day for most women and no more than two drinks a day for most men. A standard drink is defined as twelve ounces of beer, five ounces of wine, or one and one-half ounces of eighty-proof distilled spirits. These guidelines exclude people who take certain medications, are elderly, or have other health risks. Talk to your doctor about your own circumstances.

There is universal agreement that excessive alcohol consumption is bad for your heart. Even so, some people with severe heart disease or those recovering from a heart attack may be tempted to shift to heavier drinking to escape their depression or as a stress reliever. There are other heart patients who have a history of heavy drinking or destructive social drinking that need to curb their alcohol consumption altogether.

Ask yourself the Best Questions to determine if you have a drinking problem. These Best Questions were created after a review of hundreds of questions and sources, including the following respected self-assessment tools. Dr. Hanson notes that the Michigan Alcohol Screening Test (www.ncadd-sfv.org/symptoms/mast_test .html) is considered especially reliable:

1. Michigan Alcohol Screening Test (MAST)
2. Betty Ford Clinic
3. Paddington Alcohol Test
4. Alcohol Use Disorders Identification Test (AUDIT)
5. Short Alcohol Dependence Data (SADD) Questionnaire
6. National Institute on Alcohol Abuse and Alcoholism

THE QUESTION DOCTOR SAYS:

These questions are purposely in a yes/no format to simplify your self-assessment. If you have a majority of yes answers, talk to your doctor, seek professional counseling, or join a support group, such as Alcoholics Anonymous (www.aa.org).

>>> THE 10 BEST QUESTIONS
To Assess Your Drinking Habits

1. Has my drinking caused me any problems?

You define "problem." Being defensive about your drinking and hiding it from others is considered a pattern of problem behavior. Another pattern is to feel guilty about drinking or annoyed by others' criticism about it. Dr. Hanson advises, "People have trouble being objective about this topic."

2. Have I ever been in trouble because of my drinking?

This includes injuring yourself or others, angering family or friends, getting into physical fights, or drinking as much as you wanted without regard for your responsibilities the next day. Another warning sign is if you have been arrested for driving under the influence of alcohol (DUI).

3. Does my drinking worry my family or friends?

Consider whether the people who know you best and truly care about you have told you that you need to cut down. Your drinking buddies won't tell you (or know), so they don't count.

4. Has my drinking ever gotten me into trouble at work?

Examples include being frequently late for work; losing a job, business, or clients; or staying home because of drinking.

5. Do I drink alone or to relieve my feelings of anger, sadness, guilt, shyness, or lack of self-confidence?

Drinking as escapism, especially when you are alone, is an unhealthy sign.

6. Do I ever forget what I did while I was drinking?

Blackouts and memory losses are not normal. Dr. Hanson says, "You may be okay while you are drinking, but the next day you can't remember what you did. This is widely believed to be an indicator of problems."

7. Have I changed friends or started hanging out with people who are heavy drinkers?

Other versions of this question are: "Do my friends drink less alcohol than I do?" "Is drinking hurting my reputation?" "Have I ever lost friends due to drinking?" "Do I ever avoid certain people after a heavy drinking session?"

8. Do I need a drink to get going during some mornings?

Drinking before noon is a huge warning sign of problem drinking, especially the morning after an evening drinking session.

9. Do I plan my day around when and where I can drink?

Looking forward to drinking and planning your day's activities around it indicates possible alcohol dependency.

10. Has my drinking caused any medical problems?

The follow-up questions here include: "Have I ever been hospitalized because of drinking?" "Has my doctor ever told me to quit drinking?" "What did my cardiologist say about my heart's condition and drinking?"

❯ The Magic Question

Have I ever tried to cut back or quit drinking but been unsuccessful?

If you answer yes to this question, you are in essence admitting that you recognize you have a problem. Double-check your response to Best Question 1.

Now, what are you going to do about it post–heart attack or with a severe heart disease diagnosis? *You* hold the key to that answer.

CONCLUSION

Drinking is like a balancing act because alcohol is a double-edged sword. On the one hand, moderate drinkers may enjoy long-term health benefits. On the other hand, alcohol in excess can be a destructive force. Heavy drinking elevates blood pressure and increases the risk of sudden cardiac death and irregular heart rhythms (arrhythmias).

Researchers and doctors don't yet fully understand alcohol's impact on the heart. Dr. Hanson advises, "Physicians need to become very sensitive to the issues about alcohol abuse and what treatments are available. Your family physician isn't likely to be up on all the latest research."

For heart attack survivors, the experts do seem to agree that you can enjoy your daily drink or two. But be careful about drinking more as a way to fight off depression or other emotional responses to your cardiac event.

There are many available sources of help if you need it. Alcoholics Anonymous (AA) is just one. Dr. Hanson concludes, "I'd rather be addicted to AA than to alcohol. I see no problem with AA, especially if you want to quit entirely. They have groups primarily for women, Hispanics, or gays, and you can find which group is best for you."

THE 10 BEST RESOURCES

Alcoholics Anonymous. "44 Questions." www.alcoholics-anonymous.org/en_pdfs/p-2_44questions.pdf.

Alcoholics Anonymous: *The Big Book,* 4th ed. New York: Alcoholics Anonymous World Services, Inc., 2002.

Alcoholics Anonymous. "How to Find A.A. Meetings." www.alcoholics anonymous.org/en_find_meeting.cfm.

American Heart Association. "Alcohol, Wine, and Cardiovascular Disease." www.americanheart.org/presenter.jhtml?identifier=4422.

American Heart Association. "Risk Factors and Coronary Heart Disease: AHA Scientific Position." www.americanheart.org/presenter.jhtml?identifier=4726.

Hanson, David J. "Drinking Alcohol and Heart Disease: Facts & Information." www2.potsdam.edu/hansondj/healthissues/20070322142630.html.

Fletcher, Anne M. *Sober for Good: New Solutions for Drinking Problems: Advice from Those Who Have Succeeded.* New York: Houghton Mifflin, 2002.

National Institute on Alcohol Abuse and Alcoholism. "How to Cut Down on Your Drinking." http://pubs.niaaa.nih.gov/publications/handout.htm.

National Institute on Alcohol Abuse and Alcoholism. "Tips for Cutting Down on Drinking." http://pubs.niaaa.nih.gov/publications/Tips/tips.pdf.

ScienceDaily. "Light to Moderate Drinking Reduces Risk of Cardiac Events, Death." www.sciencedaily.com/releases/2006/07/060725091512.htm.

PART IV

Building Your Future Life

The last section of the book addresses the practical emotional, loving, sexual, intimate, social, and spiritual needs of heart attack survivors and heart disease patients. Each chapter offers the Best Questions to ask yourself or others as you explore your life after a heart attack or serious heart scare.

Chapter 20 offers the Best Questions to help you explore your emotional state after a heart attack, which is often quite a rollercoaster ride. In chapter 21 you'll find what you and your partner can ask each other to open up the lines of communication. There's often guilt, blame, and misunderstanding between partners following a cardiac event. This chapter provides guidance and gives you "permission" to have this difficult conversation.

Use chapter 22 to ask each other tough questions about sexual and intimate relations after one person has been diagnosed with heart disease or has had a heart attack. This chapter also tells what to ask your doctor about sex. See chapter 23 to make a well-informed decision about joining a support group, either as a heart patient or for help with smoking and alcohol consumption.

Nearly everyone can benefit from exploring their financial health in chapter 24. The 10 Worst Questions in chapter 25 are partly just for fun and also to illustrate what even well-intended friends and loved ones shouldn't (but often do) say to recovering heart patients. Chapter 26 has the Best Questions to get in deeper touch with your spiritual health after a heart attack.

The Question Doctor sincerely hopes these questions will serve as your companion and be a guiding force as you redefine the relationships in your life and strive to make peace with your broken heart.

CHAPTER 20: THE 10 BEST QUESTIONS

For Emotional Health for Heart Patients

Let's not forget that little emotions are the great captains
of our lives and we obey them without realizing it.
—Vincent Van Gogh

A heart attack is not only life-threatening but also emotionally transforming. Heart disease can be a powerful wake-up call for change and a catalyst to stop and examine your emotions, your coping skills, your relationships, and yourself.

Most survivors' initial reactions include feeling overwhelmed, shocked, angry, scared silly, confused, and oftentimes very alone or depressed. Chances are your own emotional roller-coaster ride has included all these feelings, especially depression or stress.

Typically doctors (and you) go into hyperdrive to save your life after a heart attack, and thanks to modern advances, they are often quite successful. However, your heart can still be broken—emotionally—in profound ways that can negatively impact your recovery and long-term good health.

A heart attack or a diagnosis of heart disease may darken your outlook on life. A 2008 study by the Centers for Disease Control and Prevention found that heart disease patients felt they had a lower quality of life, especially those who were women, African-American, or Hispanic. Many research studies have concluded that optimistic people tend to live longer, yet a majority of heart attack survivors report feeling depressed.

Ask yourself the following Best Questions to clarify your feelings, tap into the important mind-body connection, and hopefully

JOURNALING

When first recovering, some heart patients start a journal of everything that is happening to them—what the doctors say about their treatments and what they learn from Web sites or books about heart disease. Others prefer to keep a more reflective personal log about their feelings, relationships, spiritual thoughts or prayers, hopes, dreams, and reasons for gratitude.

If you like this idea, find your own way of journaling. Try to write something every day without self-criticism, editing, or seeing it as a chore. You can tell your story with pictures and photographs, too. For more ideas, see the Web sites CaringBridge (www.caringbridge.org) or WomenHeart (www.womenheart.org).

find peace of mind. These questions are directed at heart attack survivors but work equally well if you've been diagnosed with heart disease.

Keep in mind there's no judgment here and no right or wrong answers, only degrees of emotional honesty or dishonesty with yourself. Share with others only if you want to.

>>> THE 10 BEST QUESTIONS
For Emotional Health for Heart Patients

1. What was my emotional state before my heart attack (or diagnosis of heart disease)?

One way to recover your sense of balance is to reflect on who you were and define your emotional state before your heart attack or diagnosis. Maybe you were overstressed in a dead-end job, arguing constantly with your defiant teenager, or barely hanging on to a rocky marriage. Or life was good, full of grandchildren, church activities, and postretirement travel.

Think of this question as an emotional audit and a reality check. Be honest with yourself to avoid mourning the "good old days"— which may not have been as great as you remember.

2. What coping strategies have been most successful for me in the past?

Before now, what were your greatest emotional and personal challenges? How did you handle them? What did you do especially well and feel most proud about?

Analyze your past successes so that you can start from a position of personal strength. Get out your past coping strategies, take a look at them, shine them up, accentuate the positive, and use them again.

3. How do I feel about my physical changes?

You aren't required to like the changes you can see, like your surgery scar. It may remind you every day of that horrible moment when you had your heart attack.

But there are also emotions connected to physical changes in less obvious ways, like realizing your own vulnerability. Dr. Caela Farren, a management consultant in Virginia, recalls her 2004 heart attack: "From an emotional perspective, it was such a reversal for me after having spent my life taking care of other people. The need to be taken care of, not to be able to get out of bed, and for the first time in my life to be totally dependent, made me feel so vulnerable."

Explore your feelings about your physical changes and how these feelings may affect your self-image, self-confidence, and road to recovery. If you are truly down on yourself, it may be more difficult to make positive lifestyle changes or even to complete a cardiac rehabilitation program.

4. How well am I handling other people's reactions to my heart attack?

How other people, especially loved ones, cope with your heart attack or diagnosis affects you more than you may realize. Family members and friends can be great support sources but can also cause you additional emotional hardship and stress.

For example, if a brother freaks out and is terribly fearful for you, it's only human nature to absorb his fear and react with fear, too. Another brother may anger you because all he talks about is bad family genes and his own heart attack prospects while completely ignoring you.

Perhaps your partner is now treating you like you are made of glass and ready to break at any minute. Of course, this isn't true, but this reaction may make you feel helpless or out of control.

Others may pull away from you, blame you for your heart attack or heart disease, or act like nothing is wrong. Unexpected reactions from others can cause you to become depressed, stressed out, or angry, especially if you don't have an outlet to discuss your feelings.

5. Where can I get help? Who are my best resources for support?

Talk to your family doctor, cardiologist, support group, family, friends, or a trusted religious leader about getting help. Don't be afraid to ask for help or actively seek it out.

You deserve support and comfort as you recover from your heart attack or deal with heart disease. If you don't take care of yourself, you may jeopardize your future health and well-being.

THE QUESTION DOCTOR SAYS:

In psychiatrist Dr. Elisabeth Kübler-Ross's 1969 groundbreaking book *On Death and Dying,* she outlined five stages of grief as the pattern most people experience as they face a life-threatening illness or deal with grief:

1. **Shock and denial.** "This can't be happening to me."
2. **Anger.** "Why me? This isn't fair. I want my own life, too."
3. **Bargaining.** "Just let me live through another day."
4. **Depression.** "Why even bother anymore?"
5. **Acceptance.** "I'm going to be okay and live through this."

Not everyone moves neatly through the stages in an orderly fashion or at the same pace. For example, you might experience anger (stage 2) and then depression (stage 4), go backward to denial (stage 1), or get stuck at bargaining (stage 3).

The next five Best Questions use Dr. Kübler-Ross's stages to help you get in touch with your emotional responses to your heart condition and survival.

6. What am I denying or avoiding about my heart attack and heart disease? (Stage 1)

After a heart attack, the abstractness of death becomes more real. Dr. Daniel Forman, an assistant professor of medicine and cardiac rehabilitation expert at Harvard University, observes, "So many people deal with their fear with blatant denial. They start eating doughnuts every day as if to say, 'I didn't have a heart attack and I can eat whatever I want.'"

What matters the most is how well you face the facts that you've had a heart attack and survived, and you are now willing to take on the hard work of making lifestyle changes. Denial must be conquered before you can be successful.

7. How can I channel my anger into a positive healing experience? (Stage 2)

Nearly everyone goes through this stage. Most heart patients feel like their lives have been hijacked by their disease. How could my body betray me like this?

You may also be angry at yourself, other family members, your doctors, or God for your heart attack. Try to channel your anger into positive actions, like researching heart disease, eating better, or making overdue changes in your exercise habits.

It's very important to move beyond this stage. The people who get stuck here double their odds for having a second heart attack. Dr. Hamilton Beazley, author of the book *No Regrets,* says, "You have to look for the lessons and the gifts. But you can't do that until you get over the anger. Every tragedy brings lessons." Get professional help if your anger is out of control. Whatever you do, don't stay angry forever.

8. What am I bargaining for either consciously or unconsciously? (Stage 3)

Dr. Kübler-Ross describes this stage in her book *On Death and Dying:* "Bargaining is really an attempt to postpone; it has to include a prize offered 'for good behavior,' it also sets a self-imposed deadline . . . like children who say, 'I will never fight with my sister again.'"

Does this sound familiar? Maybe you've had fleeting thoughts of all the good things you'll do for your family or for yourself if God just lets you live. Fear is a major component of bargaining and plays a key (and unconscious) role in your choice of treatments.

Bargaining is another dangerous place to get stuck because it can lead to an endless loop of trying to do the "right" things. Failing to meet your own self-imposed overly high standards can then result in despair.

9. Why do I feel so depressed? Shouldn't I feel lucky to be alive? (Stage 4)

According to the Cleveland Clinic, one in six heart attack patients suffers from depression and up to one-half of all cases are never diagnosed. Dr. Richard Stoltz, the director for military and family health at the National Naval Medical Center in Bethesda, Maryland, comments, "The failure to acknowledge the potential difficulties of adjusting to changes can contribute to a person becoming overwhelmed."

The American Heart Association recommends that heart patients should be regularly screened for depression because it is three times more common among heart attack survivors than the general population. Lisa M. Tate, CEO of WomenHeart, an organization that provides community and online support groups for women, adds, "Many women especially suffer from depression after a heart attack." It may take you a while to sort through the complex, powerful emotions that often temporarily plague heart attack survivors and others with heart conditions.

You can move beyond depression by proactively arming yourself with medical knowledge about heart disease and healthy lifestyle changes, like how to start good exercise habits and make heart-healthy diet plans.

Seek professional help if you have suicidal thoughts, your depression persists more than two weeks, or you have no one to talk with. See also chapter 14 on coping with stress.

10. What steps can I take to accept my heart disease? (Stage 5)

Dr. Kübler-Ross believed that it's the acknowledgment of loss that holds the key to acceptance with dignity and grace. Another version of this Best Question is, "How can I treat myself with more compassion?"

Acceptance and self-love can help you overcome your internal critic who only remembers your former Big Mac habit or fondness for Snickers candy bars and Marlboro cigarettes. Guilt drains your energy to make positive changes on the road to recovery.

❯ The Magic Question

How can I feel my best today?

Many heart-disease patients allow their diagnosis, external circumstances, or other people to determine how they feel. You can take back control of your feelings with this Magic Question. It puts you in the driver's seat and makes you an active player rather than a passive victim of heart disease.

Your renewed sense of self-worth and confidence for living is priceless. Start each day with this Magic Question to find your own emotional well-being, self-acceptance, and a sense of inner peace.

CONCLUSION

Surviving a heart attack or getting a diagnosis of heart disease can flood you with complex and changing emotions that are rarely acknowledged or discussed. But they matter. Don't hesitate to ask for help. There are many resources available from your medical team, the Internet, in this book, or in other books. The bottom line is: *You are not alone.*

THE 10 BEST RESOURCES

Amen, Daniel G. *Change Your Brain, Change Your Life: The Breakthrough Program for Conquering Anxiety, Depression, Obsessiveness, Anger, and Impulsiveness.* New York: Three Rivers Press, 1998.

Blakeslee, Sandra. "HEALTH: Study Links Emotions to Second Heart Attacks." *New York Times,* September 20, 1990. http://query.nytimes.com/gst/fullpage.html?res=9C0CEEDA103DF933A1575AC0A966958260&sec=health&spon=&pagewanted=print.

Borysenko, Joan. *Minding the Body, Mending the Mind,* rev. ed. New York: Da Capo Press, 2007.

Boss, Pauline. *Ambiguous Loss: Learning to Live with Unresolved Grief.* Cambridge: Harvard University Press, 1999.

Freed, Rachael. "At the Heart of the Matter: The Emotions of the Heart." In *Heartmates: A Guide for the Spouse and Family of the Heart Patient,* 3rd ed. Minneapolis, MN: Fairview Press, 2002.

Kübler-Ross, Elisabeth. *On Grief and Grieving: Finding the Meaning of Grief Through the Five Stages of Loss.* New York: Simon & Schuster, 2005.

Mayo Clinic. "Denial: Overcome Denial by Taking Action and Moving Forward." www.mayoclinic.com/health/denial/SR00043.

Moyers, Bill. *Healing and the Mind.* New York: Main Street Books, 1995.

Sotile, Wayne, and Robin Cantor-Cooke. *Thriving with Heart Disease: A Unique Program for You and Your Family/Live Happier, Healthier, Longer.* New York: Free Press, 2003.

Williams, J. Mark G., John D. Teasdale, Zindel V. Segal, and Jon Kabat-Zinn. *The Mindful Way Through Depression: Freeing Yourself from Chronic Unhappiness.* New York: Guilford Press, 2007.

CHAPTER 21: THE 10 BEST QUESTIONS

When Talking with Your Partner After a Heart Attack

> There is no substitute for the comfort supplied by the
> utterly taken-for-granted relationship.
> —Iris Murdoch

A heart attack or diagnosis of severe heart disease will almost surely have a profound effect on your marriage or long-term partnership. A heart attack or chronic illness can magnify a relationship's past imperfections or strengthen what was already strong between partners. Rarely does a heart attack cause a divorce or separation.

But communication breakdowns can happen due to shifting roles in the partnership. The well spouse is suddenly thrust into the role of caregiver. A key difference between men and women is their comfort with the role of caregiver. Some men find this role unfamiliar and awkward because they are accustomed to solving problems. They often prefer to be Mr. Fix-it and then move on.

Daily routines can be heaved upside down, almost like an earthquake has rocked your home. Both partners feel tremendous stress, usually within their relationship as well as from external stressors, like going through surgeries, treatments, overbooked schedules, and financial worries.

The goal of this chapter is to help you and your partner communicate better by asking each other the following Best Questions. These questions will work in either direction—the heart patient asking his partner or the partner asking the patient—and will work for all couples, including gay or lesbian relationships. Revisit these

THE QUESTION DOCTOR SAYS

How you ask your questions is just as important in a close relationship as *what* you ask each other. These Best Questions give you permission to ask each other the tough questions that you might have avoided or may not have known to ask otherwise.

Your attitude and timing are critical to a successful conversation. Plan a time to talk when you are both relaxed. Use the questions in whatever order works best for you or add your own. Take a time-out when you need to or if you become upset while talking.

Here's good advice from Harriette Cole, author of the nationally syndicated advice column *Sense and Sensitivity* and the creative director of *Ebony* magazine: "It's best in the beginning to ask welcoming questions. Do your best not to be hostile, or condescending or doubting or in any way negative in your questions. . . . Ask your questions honestly and without judgment and not like an inquisition."

Best Questions over time to help you to understand how your relationship is changing and where your current needs are.

>>> THE 10 BEST QUESTIONS
When Talking with Your Partner After a Heart Attack

1. When were we most successful in communicating with each other in the past? How can we use the same methods now to deal with this illness together?

Heart disease is the newest member of your family, an uninvited houseguest who's here to stay. Your communication may be hampered by unspoken guilt or blame feelings ("If only I hadn't used so much salt in my cooking," etc.).

One way to start this conversation is to reflect on the past good times. Talk over those times and remember how well you communicated.

A MESSAGE FROM MARS AND VENUS

Dr. John Gray, relationship guru and author of the best-selling book series *Men Are from Mars, Women Are from Venus,* says, "The biggest problem between men and women is this. She gives an answer and he assumes there's a period and that's the end of the point. That's never the end of the point, she's just warming up."

Longtime partners often assume they can read each other's minds. This can be a fatal flaw and can shut down good listening. It's better to talk in specifics with frequent "I" and "we" messages ("I think we should . . . ," "I feel we need to consider . . ."). Use openers like, "I hear you saying . . . Is that right?" or "Tell me more." Keep your facial expressions open and your body language positive.

2. What areas of our lives must we maintain to ensure as much normalcy as possible?

When heart disease moves into your home, you need some semblance of normalcy in order to function on a daily basis. Solve this problem together. Your life and household responsibilities must continue, but which ones are critical needs (like paying the bills) and which ones are the "wants" (continuing your daughter's flute lessons)? The daily bottom-line question, "What's for dinner?" isn't going away during one partner's recuperation.

There's also a certain soothing aspect of normalcy. Besides practical considerations, you need normalcy in your other relationships. Keeping up by e-mail with long-distance friends, for example, might belong in your "Have to Have" bucket rather than in your "Nice to Have" bucket.

3. What role changes in our partnership do we need to make to get through this thing together?

Your past roles and the division of labor in your partnership may be turned upside down after a heart attack. In essence, you have two new job descriptions to write. This is a critical task that should not be overlooked. Couples' misunderstandings or unspoken assumptions about roles are a breeding ground for festering guilt, resentments, and even lifelong animosities toward each other.

You two need to clarify expectations soon after the heart patient comes home from the hospital. The well partner may need to cook or get take-out meals. The patient may feel her personal freedom and control are jeopardized by the very acts of kindness her partner thinks he's performing on her behalf.

Kathy Berra, MSN, the clinical director of Stanford University's Heart Network, says, "A heart attack takes a huge toll on spouses and partners. Even a year later, if the spouse says that he'll be home at 6:20 and doesn't show up until 6:40, there's that little voice in your head that says, 'Oh my God, something bad must have happened.'"

4. What has this been like for you?

This simple question may uncover a hornet's nest of complaints, a flood of feelings, or no new information at all. Heart attack survivors can get hung up on their own fragile mortality and health without fully considering their partners.

Relationship advisers Dr. Scott Peck and Shannon Peck of Solana Beach, California, comment, "There are many ways to bring the empowering combination of kindness and love into your marriage. One way is to ask simple, direct questions."

Rachael Freed, a psychotherapist and the author of the book *Heartmates,* says, "For a partner to say, 'I was terrified' is a very powerful thing. It's loving, supportive, and honest. There's shame in having a heart attack. What kind of 'manly man' would have a heart attack?"

This Best Question works at all stages of treatment and recovery, so ask it more than once.

5. How can we help each other deal with the stress in our lives?

You may be facing a double-dose stress whammy. There are tensions between you and your partner as a natural reaction to unexpected changes that are beyond your control.

Many couples experience internal misunderstandings, self-pity, misdirected anger, and financial and sexual problems after a heart attack or a diagnosis of heart disease. There are external stressors, too, such as the uncertainty of test results or the logistics of getting the heart patient to a cardiac rehab program. All of this is added to the pressure cooker of the usual work and family demands. Maryland licensed clinical social worker Mark Gorkin, says, "Caregivers frequently cycle between anger, due to the unreasonable demands of caregiving, and being in a state of chronic guilt and stress for not being able to do it all."

The only way out is to work together as a team. Identify what's causing each of you the greatest stress and then talk over what you can practically do to alleviate some of it. Some friends or family members might gladly help with routine errands or chores.

6. How can I show you that I love you?

Welcome to the "Hugs Department." There's an old saying that "hugs are the universal medicine." Even if you are still working out your needs and sex and intimacy boundaries, saying, "I love you," or giving small tokens of your affection can mean the world to a recovering heart patient or an overworked caregiver.

7. How can we still enjoy being together and have fun?

Heart disease doesn't rob you of a sense of humor. Sure, you probably can't do all the things you could before, but that doesn't mean you can't do anything that's fun or at least talk about what you will do after your recovery.

What's something silly or easy that you two can do together once in a while just like the old days? Get your favorite take-out food, watch a stupid movie together, take a walk together, or see old friends.

Being sick is no fun, but laughter can go a long way in strengthening the good glue of your relationship. See chapter 25.

8. What can I do to help you now and later?

It might just be the little things, like doing household chores or errands, or calling friends with the news about your heart attack. Or the heart patient might secretly need more reassurance despite his brave front.

The basic gender disconnect is that women don't have much practice in asking for help and men only know how to solve problems. By asking each other this question, you can talk about these differences and explore your true needs.

9. Do we need professional counseling or other help for our marriage?

It's a sign of strength to know when you need outside help to overcome your differences or communication breakdowns. There is nothing to be ashamed of if you decide you need marriage counseling, want to join a support group, or decide to meet with a therapist. When one partner is sick, it puts a tremendous burden on the relationship, even if it is a top-notch one.

10. What old rules do we need to break? What new rules do we need to establish?

Most relationships have unwritten but inviolable rules that govern everything from who takes the garbage out to how nutritious dinner has to be. This is the opposite of Best Question 2. Now we're talking about what you *do* want to change.

Your old rules are probably pretty simple, even if you've never exactly thought of them before as rules. Typically, there are rules for household chores (who does what and when), favorite routines that may need permission (Friday night poker games or shopping sprees), and the little picky stuff (neatly folded laundry or how to stack bowls in the dishwasher).

Other times rules and relationships can be complex. Some heart patients use their health to manipulate their loved ones. For example, recall Redd Foxx in the 1970s television series *Sanford and Son* as he melodramatically clutched his heart and warned his son, Lamont, "Here comes the Big One." Rachael Freed comments: "It's not unusual for the heart attack patient to control family relations later with threats like, 'Stop that or I'll have another heart attack!'"

Figure out together which rules to keep or toss to match your new circumstances. A household's unwritten and unspoken rules can be a source of unspoken assumptions and subsequent misunderstandings between partners. Call a truce on judging each other's past actions, wipe the slate clean, and start over as a team effort.

❭ The Magic Question

What are you afraid to ask me? What are we not talking about that needs to be addressed?

This is the all-important elephant-in-the-room question where everyone present is ignoring an obvious truth and not talking about something right under his or her nose.

So, what is *your* elephant? Most likely, your elephant is something you're intensely afraid of, like facing your own mortality, lost sexual intimacy, or unspoken worries about family finances.

Unacknowledged elephants have a way of just getting bigger and bigger unless you point them out and admit to their existence. This might be a hard question to ask each other. But with the right spirit of shared hopes and dreams, it can be the most liberating question you ever ask.

CONCLUSION

Many couples have not only survived a heart attack or heart disease together but have turned it into a positive and even enriching experience. In fact, most couples draw closer and join forces as allies together against their unwanted houseguest called heart disease.

Asking each other these Best Questions and any of your own questions will clear the air. Fears, stress, and anger are best extinguished by honest sharing and careful listening. Rachael Freed concludes, "Heart disease changes life for everyone in the family."

THE 10 BEST RESOURCES

American Counseling Association. "Counselor Directory." www.counseling.org/Resources/CounselorDirectory/TP/Home/CT2.aspx.

American Heart Association. "Heart of Caregiving." www.americanheart.org/presenter.jhtml?identifier=3039829.

Chapman, Gary. *The Five Love Languages: How to Express Heartfelt Commitment to Your Mate.* Chicago: Northfield Publishing, 1995.

Chilnick, Lawrence D. "The Family Impact." In *The First Year: Heart Disease: An Essential Guide for the Newly Diagnosed.* New York: Da Capo, 2008.

Family Caregiver Alliance. "Fact Sheets and Publications." www.caregiver.org/caregiver/jsp/publications.jsp?nodeid=345.

Freed, Rachael. *Heartmates: A Guide for the Spouse and Family of the Heart Patient,* 3rd ed. Minneapolis, MN: Fairview Press, 2002.

Gottman, John M. *The Relationship Cure: A 5 Step Guide to Strengthening Your Marriage, Family, and Friendships.* New York: Three Rivers Press, 2002.

Gottman, John M., and Nan Silver. *The Seven Principles for Making Marriage Work: A Practical Guide from the Country's Foremost Relationship Expert.* New York: John Wiley & Sons, Inc., 2000.

Gray, John. *Men Are from Mars, Women Are from Venus: The Classic Guide to Understanding the Opposite Sex.* New York: Harper Paperbacks, 2004.

Hendrix, Harville. *Getting the Love You Want: A Guide for Couples,* rev. ed. New York: Holt Paperbacks, 2007.

CHAPTER 22: THE 10 BEST QUESTIONS

For Sexual Health and Intimacy
After a Heart Attack

Love is the answer, but while you are waiting for the
answer, sex raises some pretty good questions.

—Woody Allen

Cardiologists say the first questions they are often asked by heart attack survivors are, "Can I have sex again?" and "When?" Survey results published in 2008 in the *Journal of Sexual Medicine* found that more than three-quarters of American men aged seventy-five to eighty-five and half of women that age are still interested in sex. Contrary to movie mythology, having sex doesn't increase your chances of a heart attack, a 2006 Australian study has found. In fact, the British Heart Foundation launched a campaign in 2007 to encourage regular sex as an antidote to a sedentary lifestyle.

However, it's imperative that you get your doctor's okay beforehand. Don't be too embarrassed to ask this common and natural question. Once you do have your doctor's blessing, you and your partner may struggle with restarting your normal sexual relations. This is where talking to each other about it can help.

As Dr. Julia Herman, executive director of the Kinsey Institute for Research in Sex, Gender, and Reproduction, says, "The value of asking questions for couples in intimate relationships is that it's a way of trying to see the other person as they are. . . . No matter how long they've been together, that's really crucial."

Asking each other the following Best Questions can help you to rebuild communication channels while you resume intimate relations. These questions also work well if you've been diagnosed with serious heart disease and now find yourself hesitating in the bedroom.

> **THE QUESTION DOCTOR SAYS:**
>
> Some sex experts say that the most potent — and most underutilized — sex tool is your voice. Asking each other these Best Questions along with your own questions can be fun, sexy, and rebuild your confidence to be together again.

〉〉〉THE 10 BEST QUESTIONS
For Sexual Health and Intimacy After a Heart Attack

1. How can we best communicate with each other about our needs for sex and intimacy?

Women tend to romanticize about sex while men have a body-centered or recreational approach. These natural differences between men and women explain why talking about sex can be tricky.

Your best communication might be using no words at all. Simple nonverbal cues, such as a "come hither" glance or wink, help to smooth misunderstandings and clarify your amorous intentions.

2. Are you comfortable being intimate again?

If you are having trouble with sexual relations or have stopped touching, this question will help you to find out why. There may be deep, unresolved issues that you need to address first.

Rachael Freed, a psychotherapist and the author of the book *Heartmates,* says, "Male heart patients respond to an emergency like a heart attack with denial. Many women as heart attack spouses respond with terror and are maybe even more depressed than their patient-husbands."

3. How can we redefine and restart our intimacy and sexual pleasure again?

If the answer to Best Question 2 was yes, do something about it. To get in the mood, try the following:

- Enjoy a romantic candlelight dinner or getaway trip.
- Offer a long sensual massage.
- Watch an erotic video together.

4. What physical changes in your body do you want me to know about?

A male heart patient may be reluctant to tell about his chest pains. A woman who has had heart surgery may feel her appearance is diminished. Older bodies may mean less natural lubrication for women or less stamina for men. This is a gentle way to approach a tough topic.

5. What can I do to please you?

If you focus on mutual pleasure, sex becomes fun again. Intimacy is proven good medicine—for both of you.

Harriette Cole, author of the nationally syndicated advice column, *Sense and Sensitivity,* and the creative director of *Ebony* magazine, says, "I think questions are very important in all relationships, especially in intimate relationships."

6. What's the craziest or funniest thing we could do to show our love for each other?

Rediscover your passion by having fun together. Put aside your worries and fears so that you can live in this moment of passion together—again.

7. Is there anything off-limits now that was okay before?

If you don't ask each other this question, your unspoken assumptions about what's acceptable and what's not can cause misunderstandings. Talk this question out without criticism or bringing up your past sexual or marital problems.

8. We agree we both have a low interest in sex right now. What can we do to get back on track?

This Best Question applies to the times that neither of you wants sexual relations. Assuming you want to try again, this question clears the air while keeping the door open for later.

9. We can't agree about having sexual relations or being intimate. How can we work it out?

Even if you've lost sexual desire, you can still be intimate and show affection through kissing, touching, stroking, cuddling, hugging, and massaging each other, or by sharing loving words of comfort and hope.

10. Do we need professional help?

Consider the option of talking with a professional therapist or marriage counselor. Unresolved sexual tensions can result in emotional strain and distance in long-term relationships.

❯ The Magic Question

What sexual fears are we not talking about that need to be addressed?

Not talking about sexual problems puts a tremendous strain on your relationship, just at the very time when you need closeness, good communication, and each other more than ever.

CONCLUSION

Sex may have been the last thing on your mind after your heart attack or diagnosis of heart disease— or the first thing on your mind. Being intimate can make you feel loved and supported as you cope with your illness and recovery.

THE 10 BEST RESOURCES

American Heart Association. "Sex and Heart Disease." Order information at www.americanheart.org/presenter.jhtml?identifier=9239.

American Heart Association. "Sexual Activity and Heart Disease or Stroke." www.americanheart.org/presenter.jhtml?identifier=4714.

British Heart Foundation. "Sex and Heart Disease." www.bhf.org.uk/living_with_heart_conditions/rehabilitation/sex_and_heart_disease.aspx.

Chapunoff, Eduardo, and Arnold A. Lazarus. *Answering Your Questions About Heart Disease and Sex.* Long Island City, NY: Hatherleigh Press, 2007.

Cleveland Clinic. "Heart Failure and Sexual Relationships." http://my.clevelandclinic.org/disorders/Heart_Failure/hic_Heart_Failure_and_Sexual_Relationships.aspx.

Heart and Stroke Foundation (Canada). "Intimate Relationships." www.heartandstroke.com/site/c.ikIQLcMWJtE/b.3484213/k.6149/Intimate_relationships.htm.

Heart Healthy Living. "Sex After a Heart Attack." www.hearthealthyonline.com/heart-attack-stroke/heart-attack-stroke-basics/sex-after-heart-attack_1.html.

MedicineNet. "After a Heart Attack: Can You Have Sex?" www.medicinenet.com/script/main/art.asp?articlekey=51133.

Stratmann, Henry G., and Maryellen Stratmann. *Sex and Your Heart Health: A Cardiologist Tells All.* Springfield, MO: Starship Press, 2007.

WebMD. "Sex After a Heart Attack." www.webmd.com/heart-disease/features/sex-after-a-heart-attack.

CHAPTER 23: THE 10 BEST QUESTIONS
Before Joining a Support Group

A single arrow is easily broken, but not ten in a bundle.
—Japanese proverb

Why join a support group? Because people in support groups understand; they've been there, done that, or are just learning how to cope with severe heart disease, survive a heart attack, or quit smoking or drinking just like you are. Where else could you find a banker and a construction worker sharing their personal stories with each other?

A support group is defined as a group of people who meet on a regular basis with a trained group leader to discuss their concerns and feelings about the disease they have in common, such as heart disease, addiction to smoking, or alcoholism. There are also moderated and nonmoderated online support groups that are similar except the people involved rarely meet in person.

All support groups seek to help to restore your self-confidence, connect with a community of understanding people, and learn more about your disease or condition. People of all races and backgrounds come to support groups to find an outlet for their similar worries and issues as a result of living with a chronic illness. The advantages of belonging to a support group include:

- Connecting with others who are going through the same thing
- Overcoming feelings of isolation, fear, and being overwhelmed
- Getting insider information on the best doctors, treatments, books, and Web sites

- Expressing confusing or frightening emotions in a safe environment
- Feeling less helpless and knowing where to get more help
- Giving loved ones touched by this disease (partner, family, and friends) an outlet, too

Sometimes support groups are associated with formal cardiac rehabilitation programs. Dr. Larry F. Hamm, president of the American Association of Cardiovascular and Pulmonary Rehabilitaion and a cardiac specialist at The George Washington University, suggests, "There's often a built-in support group from the cardiac rehab experience." If so, take advantage of it.

Dr. Daniel Forman, an assistant professor at Harvard Medical School, agrees. He says, "I think it's both men and women that need support groups. They are an important human dimension in cardiac recovery." Lisa Tate, the CEO of WomenHeart, a support group for women who have had a cardiac event, adds, "It's all about making a connection with other women who have heart disease but are managing to live quality lives anyway."

Ask the group leader or online moderator the following Best Questions to learn more about a support group before joining it.

>>>THE 10 BEST QUESTIONS
Before Joining a Support Group

1. Who leads the group? What is this person's background, formal training, and experience with people who have heart disease or my diagnosis?

A skillful and experienced group leader can make a huge difference in your enjoyment and benefits from a support group. Look for someone who has already gone through heart disease, smoking ces-

THE QUESTION DOCTOR SAYS:

Find out how this group leader deals with confidentiality issues. You may be sensitive and not want your personal situation discussed outside of the support group.

sation, or alcohol withdrawal himself. The ideal group leader or facilitator also has training in managing group dynamics and emotions.

2. What does the group talk about?

The best support groups share common problems, fears, knowledge, and humor. You want a sense of community and a warm atmosphere that welcomes all comers and comments without criticism or judgment.

3. Which types of heart disease (or other medical conditions) are the participants dealing with?

If you have choices, you might want a support group where all the participants share the same problems. For example, if you've had a heart attack caused by coronary artery disease, you may not relate to someone born with a congenital heart defect.

4. Are the participants either heart patients or family members, or are both in a mixed group?

Again, this question may not matter to you or you may have limited choices. Just be aware that people with early heart disease may be less sympathetic to older people who have survived a heart attack—and vice versa.

5. What is the size and turnover of the group?

Lively discussions happen when groups have between six and fifteen attendees. People often drift in and out of support groups, depending on their other activities and responsibilities.

If you want more long-term stability, look for a well-established group of soul mates. It will save you from having to retell your story and meet new people at each meeting.

6. Do any of the support group members socialize at times besides the regular group meetings?

You may not care about extended friendships outside of the support group. Just be aware of your own preferences ahead of time so that you don't feel either forced or neglected by the other group members.

7. Who is sponsoring the group and why?

Most support groups are sponsored by nonprofit groups, hospitals, medical associations, and other community or religious-based organizations. Be just a little more wary of online groups until you know more about who's behind them and what, if any, hidden motives they may have, such as promoting new heart drugs or seeking volunteers to participate in a clinical trial.

8. Where does the group hold its meetings?

Face-to-face groups meet in hospital settings, members' homes, churches, community centers, and other public locations. The convenience of the support group's location is likely to be important to you as well as its general ambience (an impersonal hospital setting versus someone's living room).

9. Is there an online component?

There are thousands of people in online groups discussing heart disease, smoking or drinking cessation, and other medical conditions. Some groups chat on specific issues, like treatments or side effects, while others have less direction and structure. For example, Lorraine Biros, client services director of the Mautner Project, the National Lesbian Health Organization, suggests, "It's important for lesbian patients to find a lesbian support group."

10. What other alternatives to face-to-face support group meetings do I have?

You may need help beyond a support group's capability. If so, seek private counseling with a therapist, social worker, or trusted religious or community leader. See chapters 20 and 21 on emotions and partner relationships.

❯ The Magic Question

How does the group leader protect participants' emotions and egos during group discussions?

There are certain risks to being an active member of a support group and sharing your true thoughts and feelings. A first-class group facilitator creates a safe place for people to share their stories and personal vulnerabilities.

The use of ground rules for discussion, such as, "All comments are welcome, but no personal attacks," defines the boundaries of acceptable discussion topics and behaviors and creates a safety net for all participants.

CONCLUSION

Seeking a support group may be the healthiest thing you can do for yourself, even if you usually aren't a "group person" or can think of a million excuses. The American Lung Association's national program manager for smoking cessation, Bill Blatt, says, "Even if you aren't a 'support group person,' try it out anyway. You'll be with other people who are going through exactly the same thing and they can offer advice and help you be successful. Support groups are generally very helpful."

THE 10 BEST RESOURCES

Alcoholics Anonymous. "How to Find A.A. Meetings. www.aa.org/lang/en/subpage.cfm?page=28.

American Cancer Society. "Choosing a Support Group." www.cancer.org/docroot/ESN/ESN_1.asp?sitearea=ESN.

American Cancer Society. "How to Find Online Support Groups." www.cancer.org/docroot/ESN/content/ESN_1_4X_How_to_Find_Online_Support_Groups.asp?sitearea=ESN.

American Heart Association. "Forum: Heart Failure." http://my.americanheart.org/jiveforum/forum.jspa?forumID=16.

American Heart Association. "Local Information." www.americanheart.org/presenter.jhtml?identifier=3005688.

American Lung Association. "Search by State." www.lungusa.org/site/apps/kb/zip/zip.asp?c=dvLUK9O0E&b=37083.

Cleveland Clinic. "Support Groups and Organizations." http://my.clevelandclinic.org/heart/education/supportgroups.aspx.

Inspire. "Heart and Circulation Groups." www.inspire.com/categories/heart-and-circulation.

Mended Hearts. "Membership." www.mendedhearts.org/frame-education.htm.

WomenHeart. "WomenHeart Bulletin Board." www.womenheart.org/bulletin_board.asp.

CHAPTER 24: THE 10 BEST QUESTIONS

For a Heart Patient's Financial Health

> Money makes a good servant, but a bad master.
>
> —Francis Bacon

As a heart patient, you probably face financial challenges that may not have even occurred to you yet. Chronic heart disease not only affects your health but also your wallet.

Every situation is different. Perhaps you've been the main breadwinner of your family and now you can't go back to work for a while. Maybe you were ready to retire anyway or have other income.

Health Day News reports that seventy-nine million Americans said they had trouble paying off their medical bills and debts in 2007. If this sounds familiar, your financial difficulties won't be solved easily. But having a heart-to-heart talk with yourself is a great first step. Think of your heart troubles as a wake-up call to get more financially savvy.

The following Best Questions are written for heart patients and their families. This chapter should not be used as a substitute for professional financial or tax advice.

>>> THE 10 BEST QUESTIONS
For a Heart Patient's Financial Health

1. How well organized are my/our personal financial papers, accounts, and records?

Managing financial records and bills is a challenge for most people. You may resist the tedious task of creating filing systems. But care-

THE QUESTION DOCTOR SAYS:

Start your financial discussions early. Having these discussions now, even if they are hard, can result in a concrete action plan to deal with troubling situations before they become crises.

These Best Questions are also useful as the foundation for family meetings on finances. Many families believe advanced planning reduces their stress because they feel more in control and make better-informed decisions.

ful financial planning starts with putting financial documents in one place and taming any "clutter monsters" lurking under your bed. Important financial and legal documents include:

- Bank and brokerage account information
- Birth certificates
- Deeds, mortgage papers, and ownership statements
- Passwords, account numbers, and safety deposit access
- Insurance policies
- Monthly or outstanding bills
- Pension and other retirement benefit summaries
- Rental income paperwork
- College scholarship and grant money forms for your children
- Social security information
- Stock and bond certificates

2. What are my/our financial assets?

A **financial asset** is anything you own that has monetary value. Financial assets generally refer to paper assets like accounts and funds as well as tangible property, including house ownership and the vehicles sitting in your driveway. When you are writing down all your assets, don't forget these:

- Home and real estate holdings
- 401(k) accounts
- IRAs
- Mutual funds
- Stocks and bonds
- Employee stock options
- College savings
- Other savings
- Insurance policies
- Cash
- Cars, trucks, boats, and motorcycles
- Other valuables, such as appraised collectibles, antiques, and personal property

3. What are my/our debts and expenses?

Creating and living within a budget is a necessary evil. Norman Berk, a certified financial planner in Birmingham, Alabama, comments, "A budget can help keep you out of debt as well as provide for a means to reduce existing debt. It also can be the focal point for serious review of expenditures so a plan can be developed to have the extra funds if they are suddenly necessary."

Start by identifying how you've spent your money in the past. Your debts may already be under control, but chances are they are less than ideal. Be aware that unexpected medical bills are one of the most common causes of personal bankruptcies. Include the following debts and expenses on your list:

- Mortgage payment or rent

- Credit card payments
- Auto loans
- Personal loans
- Child care expenses or child support payments
- Insurance costs
- Living expenses including food, clothing, utilities, fuel, transportation, parking, cable and Internet charges, personal care, routine doctor, dentist, and drug costs, entertainment, holiday gifts, vacations, hobbies, home repair, taxes, school tuition, magazine/newspaper subscriptions, and other miscellaneous costs

Get your FICO score if you don't already know it. A FICO score is based on your credit history and is widely used to determine if you are a good credit risk. FICO scores (an acronym for the Fair Isaac Corporation at www.myfico.com) range from a low of 300 to a perfect 850 score.

Don't go nuts over this exercise, but don't skip it either. The more you understand your current financial status, the better prepared you'll be for any new medical bills.

4. What is my/our health insurance coverage for treatments and other medical bills?

Heart disease can be costly. Many people have a portion of their medical expenses paid by their health insurance plan. If you don't, financial assistance resources are available, including government-sponsored services and voluntary programs.

If you are covered through your employer, get a copy of your policy now and familiarize yourself with coverage details. Take insurance cards to all appointments.

To sidestep costly surprises, talk to your doctor or health-care facility and your insurance carrier about your insurance coverage.

Try to get a clear idea of what your out-of-pocket costs will be, although exact amounts may be difficult to know in advance. Don't end up in insurance limbo land or the poorhouse.

5. Do I want to be temporarily off from work, retire, or continue working? What benefits and time-off flexibility can I reasonably expect from my employer?

Beyond your doctors' recommendations about working, you may have some options. Some people devote their full-time energies to healing and avoid their stressful workplaces, while others relish work as a welcome distraction from their health problems. Many people retire at this point.

For others, the need to keep their income drives all else. You may be compelled to work in order to pay medical bills and other looming debts.

Keep in mind that the Family and Medical Leave Act allows most workers in the United States twelve weeks of leave each year for a serious illness such as heart disease. You don't necessarily have to take all your leave at once.

6. Do I/we have a designated financial power of attorney? A medical power of attorney? A legally binding document stating who this person is?

Taking care of this business is hard. You may imagine your death. But think of these legal protections as an act of generosity and kindness for your loved ones. You are relieving them of the burden of making difficult decisions later.

According to Chicago-based certified financial planner Cicily Carson Maton, "A power of attorney for health is very important to have in place so your agent can pay your bills and take care of your affairs. It is absolutely vital."

A medical power of attorney is a separate but similar document that specifies your wishes if you become medically incapacitated. Consider getting this document prepared before any surgeries or long-distance travel for treatments. Your hospital or clinic may provide this form for free, but check with a lawyer or financial planner for a final blessing.

7. Do I/we have an estate plan, a will, and a living will? Are my/your/our other legal affairs in order?

Estate planning is the orderly process of preparing to transfer your affairs and assets to your intended beneficiaries. A good estate plan should also minimize taxes, court costs, and attorney's fees, while addressing your welfare and needs. Most adults need an estate plan regardless of the size of their estate.

A **will** is not just for rich people. No matter how much you have, a will helps to ensure that your children and other beneficiaries will not suffer undue confusion or anxiety about your wishes.

A **living will** (also called a **living trust** or **medical directive**) gives you the opportunity to declare your intentions about lifesaving efforts on your behalf and to appoint a representative to ensure your intentions are followed.

8. What are my/our insurance options?

Look at all your insurance, including health care coverage, Medicare, Medicaid, disability, long-term care, veterans' benefits, and life insurance plans. Understanding these policies now can save you time and money later.

A primary concern is your health insurance. Norman Berk says, "One of your early questions should be what your health insurance coverage is and its portability. Once you know what you are faced with, you need an understanding from your insurance company on what it does or doesn't cover. This will impact your other decisions."

9. What are my/our options and eligibility for government assistance programs or other assistance in paying medical bills?

The primary government health-care program for people age sixty-five and older is Medicare. Other government assistance programs include:

- Social Security Disability Income (SSDI)
- Supplemental Security Income (SSI). See www.ssa.gov/dib plan/dqualify5.htm
- Veterans' benefits. See www.vba.va.gov/VBA
- Tax deductions and credits
- Care credit

SSDI is for workers under age sixty-five who can prove an inability to work. SSI guarantees a monthly income for people age sixty-five or older, disabled, and with limited income. See www .socialsecurity.gov for more information.

Medicaid pays for medical care for very low-income people with no other resources. Veterans may qualify for health and long-term-care benefits. There are also various tax and care credits available. Check with www.benefitscheckup.org and the financial assistance organizations listed in the resource sections of this book.

10. Do I/we need help from a professional financial adviser?

Investigate services and costs before answering this question. Look for a certified financial planner with proven experience in dealing with chronically ill patients.

As you are calling around, ask for the advisers' specific services; if they sell products (be wary); their personal philosophy on financial planning (conservative, aggressive, etc.); who exactly you'll be working with; if charges are by the hour, flat fees, or commissions; and a written list of services and charges.

Paul Yurachek, a certified financial planner with Ameriprise Financial Services, says, "When people are aging, it creates a whole new set of issues, especially if there's a spouse involved. As financial advisers, we try to alleviate their concerns about money."

Financial planner Cicily Carson Maton advises, "If you didn't have any financial planning in place or have a financial adviser prior to your diagnosis, reach out to those people around you that you trust and ask for their help."

❯ The Magic Question

How can I/we avoid letting heart disease ruin my/our financial health?

This question is aimed at another potential threat to your financial stability—you.

You do have some control. Find ways to cut back on expenses and clarify your priorities. Look at your spending habits as honestly as possible. Here are some red flags from the National Foundation for Credit Counseling for poor money management:

- Always late with bill payments
- Withdrawn funds from retirement or savings accounts to pay current expenses
- Calls from creditors about overdue bills
- Credit card cash advances to pay off other creditors
- Minimum repayments on installment charges
- Overtime work to make ends meet

CONCLUSION

No matter what your financial, insurance, and employment circumstances are, you can deal with them more proactively if you take the time now to assess your situation and figure out how to locate financial assistance if needed.

When that's done, you can really focus your energies on getting well. You won't be trying to fight financial fatigue and insurance exhaustion at the same time you are healing your broken heart.

THE 10 BEST RESOURCES

Healthwell Foundation. "Helping Patients Afford Medical Treatments." Healthwell Foundation. www.healthwellfoundation.org/index.aspx.

H.E.L.P. "Financial Issues." www.help4srs.org/finance/finintro.htm.

Landay, David S. *Be Prepared: The Complete Financial, Legal and Practical Guide for Living with a Life-Challenging Condition.* New York: St. Martin's Press, 1998.

Medicare. "State Health Insurance Assistance Program." www.medicare .gov/contacts/static/allStateContacts.asp.

MetLife Mature Market Institute. "Medicare and Medicaid Programs— The Basics." www.metlife.com/FileAssets/MMI/MMISYCMedicareand Medicaid2007.pdf.

National Council on Aging. "Benefits Checkup." Searchable program at www.benefitscheckup.org.

Patient Access Network Foundation. "How to Apply." https://www .patientaccessnetwork.org/HowApply.aspx.

Patient Advocate Foundation. "Resources for Solving Insurance and Healthcare Problems." Patient Advocate Foundation. www.patientadvo cate.org.

PhRMA. "Partnership for Prescription Assistance." https://www.pparx .org/Intro.php.

Social Security Administration. "Social Security Handbook." www.ssa .gov/OP_Home/handbook/ssa-hbk.htm.

CHAPTER 25: THE 10 *WORST* QUESTIONS
To Ask a Heart Patient

Mirth is God's medicine.

—Henry Ward Beecher

After a heart attack, you have good reason to be sad, stressed, or depressed. In contrast, humor is a powerful ally. Over the past decades, studies have found that humor can reduce physical pain and stress. The message is simple: Humor is healing. The medicinal power of laughter can fight your fear and lighten your heart's load.

Patty Wooten of Santa Cruz, California, is an experienced cardiac nurse. She says, "Some emotions have a toxic effect on the body, like anger, hostility, stress, hopelessness, and depression. When we live with these emotions all the time, they create chemical changes in the body that actually weaken the immune system. Humor and laughter change our emotional state. For the moments of laughter, there are feelings of delight and joy, so we break the negative cycle. The other powerful thing about humor is that once you start to laugh, you feel more in control."

In his pioneering 1979 book, *Anatomy of an Illness,* Norman Cousins asserts that "laughter therapy" cured him from a supposedly irreversible disease. Cousins discovered while watching old Marx Brothers films and television's *Candid Camera* shows that ten minutes of belly laughs helped him sleep pain-free for two hours.

Welcome to the Hall of Shame, the Worst Questions asked by well-meaning but clueless friends and family members. These awful questions come from people who don't know what else to say

---

THE QUESTION DOCTOR SAYS:

How well does your sense of humor protect you from heart disease? Find out by taking the humor questionnaire by cardiologist Dr. Michael Miller, director of the Center for Preventive Cardiology at the University of Maryland Medical Center. See the Web site: www.umm.edu/news/releases/humor_survey.htm.

---

to a heart patient. Thanks to Patty Wooten and the heart attack survivors who contributed to this list.

>>> THE 10 *WORST* QUESTIONS
To Ask a Heart Patient

1. Will your next heart attack kill you?
Talk about insensitive questions!

2. Since you're out of commission now, can I have the rest of your Viagra?
Talk about opportunistic questions!

3. How long did the doctor give you to live?
Talk about pessimistic questions!

4. Can you blow yourself up with your nitroglycerin pills?
Talk about explosive questions! Nitroglycerin is a common treatment for heart disease *and* it is the explosive component in dynamite. Guess the question asker is hoping for some entertaining fireworks with your spontaneous human combustion.

5. Have you reserved another heart in case your next heart attack blows this one?
Answer: "Yes, and I'm looking forward to Valentine's Day, thank you."

6. When your heart stopped and you were dead for a while, did you go to heaven or hell?

Death. Been there. Done that.

7. Did I tell you about the guy I know who survived his heart attack and then dropped dead six months later?

A common and universally despised Worst Question is a long shaggy dog story about someone else's tragic ending. Maybe the listener is trying to relate to you or maybe she's just trying to one-better your story. Either way, your own heart attack story gets hijacked.

8. What did you do to cause your heart attack?

Well, okay, most heart attacks are partially because the person didn't live a lily white life, free of all temptations and naughtiness, but who's perfect? Some cardiologists believe that nearly every adult on the planet has some degree of coronary artery disease.

9. Should you be eating that?

Coming from the right person with the right tone of voice, this question shows concern for your health. But if your overbearing father-in-law who just ran the Marine Marathon in record time asks you, chances are you have a self-appointed fitness freak looking over your shoulder and watching every bite.

10. How often do you have to jumpstart your pacemaker?

Just hook your pacemaker up to the car battery and you're good to go for another fifty thousand miles.

❯ The Magic Question

How does my five-year-old grandson describe my heart condition?

Well, you're awfully old, but at least you aren't dead yet. I can still hear your heart beating.

CONCLUSION

Dr. Michael Miller's research into laughter as authentic heart medicine concluded that people with heart disease were 40 percent less likely to laugh in a variety of situations than comparable people without heart disease. Laughter as an alternative medicine for your ailing heart is no joke.

THE 10 BEST RESOURCES

Allen Klein.com. "Humor and Healing—Related Links." www.allen klein.com/links.htm.

Association for Applied and Therapeutic Humor. "AATH e-Zine." www .aath.org/ezine/ezine-2008_02.html.

Buckman, Elcha. *The Handbook of Humor: Clinical Applications in Psychotherapy.* Malabar, FL: Krieger Publishing, 1994.

The Humor Project. "Humor Sourcebook." www.humorproject.com/ publications/sourcebook.pdf.

Jest for the Health of It! "Resources/Reading List." www.jesthealth.com.

Klein, Allen. *The Courage to Laugh.* New York: Tarcher/Putnam Books, 1998.

Mullinax, Earl. *Having a Heart Attack and Keeping Your Sense of Humor.* Mustang, OK: Tate Publishing, 2006.

Neuharth, Dan. *Secrets You Keep from Yourself: How to Stop Sabotaging Your Happiness.* New York: St. Martin's Press, 2004.

Wooten, Patty. *Compassionate Laughter: Jest for Your Health,* 2nd ed. Santa Cruz, CA: JestHealth. 2000.

Wooten, Patty. Jest for the Health of It. "Articles by Patty Wooten." www .jesthealth.com/frame-articles.html.

CHAPTER 26: THE 10 BEST QUESTIONS

For Spiritual Health for Heart Patients

Courage is fear that has said its prayers.

—Dorothy Bernard, actress

A heart attack ignites a spiritual crisis for many cardiac patients and their loved ones. Some people find their belief in God shaken to the core. Others find deeper meaning in their chosen faith.

Spirituality is defined here as a general awareness of a force greater than the individual self. Religion is only one aspect of spirituality. In this holistic definition, spirituality can also mean connecting with nature, holding unspoken beliefs, or finding peace of mind in the back row of a yoga class. Dr. Christina Puchalski, the director of The George Washington University's Institute for Spirituality and Health, defines spirituality as "that part of us which gives us the ultimate meaning in life." A "faith community" is used here to broadly mean any group of people who share the same beliefs.

While there is no proof that spirituality or prayers can cure disease, many studies have shown the importance of faith in healing. Prayer can reduce your stress, anxiety, and depression, promote a more positive outlook, and strengthen your will to live. A ten-year study by the U.S. Office of Technology Assessment found an 83 percent positive effect on physical health. Another set of studies measuring spirituality's benefits concluded that 92 percent of the patients reported positive benefits.

As Dr. Puchalski observes, "Healing is more than just a cure. It's how people see themselves. You can see yourself as broken or

THE QUESTION DOCTOR SAYS:

Pace yourself as you ask yourself these Best Questions. In order to be fully reflective of each question, you may prefer to ponder them over the course of a few weeks or months. Perhaps one question per day will work for you.

Ask your own Best Questions as well. You may also choose to discuss these questions with your loved ones or faith community.

you can see yourself as a whole person who is not succumbing to this illness."

Ask yourself the following Best Questions as you explore your own spiritual journey during your recovery. Dr. Hamilton Beazley, scholar and author of the book *No Regrets,* believes, "Best Questions are like a set of physical exercises to keep the body in tune, except these questions keep us spiritually healthy."

>>>THE 10 BEST QUESTIONS
For Spiritual Health for Heart Patients

1. How important is spiritual faith or religion in my life?

A major cardiac event often results in a reassessment of the importance of your spiritual life. Some people may deny their faith and question how God could let something this bad happen to them. They may develop private doubts, skepticism, cynicism, or a sense of hollowness. For others, their heart attack translates into a reaffirmation of their faith in a new or deeper way.

No matter what your previous connection has been to your faith, you may instantly know your answer to this question or you may need to ponder it long and hard. Either way, it's your starting point for considering your spiritual health.

2. Am I angry at God because I had a heart attack? If so, how can I make peace with Him?

People who have actively practiced their religious faith, regularly attended religious services, and tried to be a "good" person may feel a terrible sense of unfairness. You may lash out and ask, "Why are You punishing me?" "What kind of God are you?"

Dr. Hamilton Beazley says, "Sometimes you have to forgive God. The anger ties you to the past. It means you aren't free." If you can't get beyond the hurt or anger, seek professional counseling so that your emotions won't cripple your heart's recovery.

Albert Einstein once said, "God may be subtle, but He isn't plain mean."

3. What role do I want my faith or religious beliefs to play in my battle against heart disease?

People have used prayer and other spiritual practices for thousands of years as tools for healing. A 2004 study by the National Center for Complementary and Alternative Medicine found that 45 percent of the people surveyed have used prayer to relieve symptoms of their illness.

Your faith may be a source of strength and comfort, may serve as a guiding force for making tough decisions, or may serve as a light at the end of the tunnel called "uncertainty." Some estranged couples or families touched by heart disease find that their shared faith keeps their communication lifeline open during tough times.

4. What support did I find in the past from my faith community?

Many people describe themselves as spiritual but don't participate in any formal religious institution or rituals. Whether your faith is connected to Christianity, Judaism, Buddhism, Islam, or Mother Nature, consider how much you have experienced comfort from your past associations with other people in your faith community.

What has been the nature of your prayers in the past? How did you respond to the past challenges in your life when you turned to your faith for comfort and hope? Who and what helped you the most?

5. How can I reconnect with my faith community to find new meaning?

A Gallup Poll in 2001 found that 43 percent of Americans attended religious services at least once a week. Sometimes people's childhood religious affiliations slip away or are consciously abandoned in adulthood. A heart attack may reawaken your need to be part of the faith community of your choice again. As workplace stress consultant Anna Maravelas observes, "Heart attacks serve as spiritual wake-up calls for many."

In addition to offering a close-knit and supportive environment, some faith communities host discussion groups or provide financial support for those with life-threatening illnesses.

6. How much do I want to share my spirituality or religious beliefs with my loved ones?

Some people believe their spirituality is a private affair and choose not to share it with even their closest loved ones. Others wouldn't dream of excluding their loved ones from their beliefs and active religious observances.

Part of this deeper quest is deciding how much of your spirituality and religious beliefs you want to be public and how much you want to be private.

7. How can my faith or religious beliefs give me the additional strength and courage that I need right now?

Your heart attack may have seemed like your darkest hour. Chances are you are facing a newly redefined life that includes many lifestyle and medical challenges that may seem daunting right now. You may see your faith or religion as your "rock of Gibraltar," a steadfast light to guide you and your loved ones during the future uncertainties and changes ahead of you.

Dr. Herbert Benson, mind-body pioneer and author of the classic book *The Relaxation Response,* says, "Frequently a person will choose a prayer to repeat as a way to quiet the mind and as an automatic linkage to spirituality. When people evoke the Relaxation Response, even using secular terms, they feel more spiritual. This is called the 'Faith Factor.'"

8. What would Jesus (or another role model) have done if He had had a heart attack?

Thinking of a role model, either a great spiritual teacher like Jesus, Buddha, or Muhammad, or a sweet spiritual person in your life, like a favorite rabbi, aunt, or former priest, is like having a mentor on call. Ask yourself what this person would do in your situation.

This isn't to suggest that you are "channeling" the spirits or some other hocus-pocus, but rather you are tapping into the wisdom that knowing this person has given you. Let that other person's strength be your anchor and companion.

Your spiritual guide can be a trusted family member or other loved one. As Dr. Puchalski says, "What people are really looking for is someone who can just be with them without trying to fix their problem, just help them get through this time."

9. What lessons does God want me to learn from my heart attack?

A heart attack may lead you to search for new meaning. You may feel compelled to ask the ultimate biggest and Best Questions of life: "Who am I?" "Why am I here?" "What does my life mean?"

Most of us rarely acknowledge our mortality. But surviving a heart attack means you have already looked your mortality straight in the eye. Now you may be ready to strengthen your relationship with God.

Perhaps His lessons for you will be profound or involve new joy in simple daily pleasures. Whatever your lessons, asking this Best Question will help you on the path of accepting what has happened.

10. Do I want my doctors to address faith issues during my health care? If so, what are my expectations?

This may not be an option if your doctors favor a clinical approach to care. Not all doctors have soft sides or open personalities. And perhaps you would be uncomfortable talking with them about faith or don't have enough time during office visits.

Dr. Betty Ferrell, RN, a clinician and research scientist in pain management at City of Hope National Medical Center in Duarte, California believes, "Pain has a spiritual and existential dimension and to ignore that is to damage the essence of the patient."

Some heart patients discover an overlooked opportunity to connect with their doctors in a deeper way than previously imagined. The key is clarifying your own expectations in advance about what role, if any, your doctor has here.

❯ The Magic Question

What unmet needs do I have concerning my faith or spirituality?

Regardless of how frequently you practice your faith or pray, you may benefit from coming to grips now with any past regrets or missed opportunities that have bothered you. For example, there may be a faith-based ritual, such as a baptism or church-blessed wedding, which you feel is overdue. Perhaps your heart attack or heart disease diagnosis will prompt you to reach out to a long-estranged parent, sibling, son, or old friend.

Surviving a heart attack is a watershed event for most people. It can also bring about a true reordering of life's priorities. Spiritual healing can be a powerful component in your journey to better health and quality of life.

CONCLUSION

"Ask and it will be given to you; seek and you will find; knock and the door will be opened to you. For everyone who asks receives; he who seeks finds; and to him who knocks, the door will be opened." (Matthew 7:7–8)

THE 10 BEST RESOURCES

American Academy of Family Physicians. "Spirituality and Health." http://familydoctor.org/online/famdocen/home/articles/650.html.

Beazley, Hamilton. *No Regrets: A Ten-Step Program for Living in the Present and Leaving the Past Behind.* Hoboken, NJ: John Wiley & Sons, 2004.

The Bible, King James version.

Chopra, Deepak. *Healing the Heart: A Spiritual Approach to Reversing Coronary Artery Disease.* Nevada City, CA: Harmony, 1998.

The George Washington University Institute for Spirituality and Health. "The Role of Spirituality in Health and Illness." www.gwish.org/slide1.ppt#260,1.

Open Directory Project. "Religion and Spirituality." www.dmoz.org/Society/Religion_and_Spirituality.

Spiritual Experiences. "Spiritual Experiences and Spirituality." www.spiritual-experiences.com.

Tolle, Eckhart. *A New Earth: Awakening to Your Life's Purpose.* New York: Penguin, 2008.

University of Minnesota's Center for Spirituality and Healing. "Home Page." www.csh.umn.edu.

Wikipedia. "Spirituality." http://en.wikipedia.org/wiki/Spirituality.

CONCLUSION: LIVING WELL WITH
HEART DISEASE

You, interrupted. That's what happens when you have a heart attack. It changes your life forever.

Heart disease is a silent and deadly killer. More than seven hundred thousand people died from heart disease in the United States last year. Forty-seven percent of people who had heart attacks didn't live to ask any more questions.

But you have. You are a survivor. As Harvard University's Dr. Daniel Forman says, "The real heroes of this story are the patients and what they do every day to organize their lives in a healthier way."

Knowledge truly is power. Asking Best Questions is your secret weapon because it empowers you to take charge of your health again.

Think of this book as the start of a lifetime of asking your own Best Questions about everything. "Being smart" has a new definition. It's not what you know. It's what you *ask* that really matters.

A good mind knows the right questions, but a great mind knows the right questions. You, recharged.

Bibliography

We regret any errors or omissions on this resource list. Inclusion on this list does not imply endorsement by the publisher or the author. We defined "best resource" as the most practical and content-rich information available with an emphasis on question lists and free online access.

THE 10 VERY BEST RESOURCES

American Heart Association. "Patient Information Sheets." www.americanheart.org/presenter.jhtml?identifier=3004356.

American Heart Association. "Questions to Ask Your Healthcare Professional." www.americanheart.org/presenter.jhtml?identifier=105.

British Heart Foundation. "Heart Information Booklets." www.bhf.org.uk/living_with_heart_conditions/patient_support_resources/heart_information_booklets.aspx.

CardioSmart. "Learn About Heart Disease." www.cardiosmart.org/HeartDisease/CTTBrowser.aspx.

Cleveland Clinic. "Heart and Vascular Institute: Resources for Patients." http://my.clevelandclinic.org/heart/guide.aspx.

Healthfinder.gov. (Provides links for 1,500 organizations and publications.) www.healthfinder.gov.

MedicineNet. "Heart Center." www.medicinenet.com/heart/focus.htm.

MedlinePlus. "Heart Diseases." www.nlm.nih.gov/medlineplus/heartdiseases.html#cat5.

National Institutes of Health. "PubMed Central." Portal to a free digital archive of medical journals. www.pubmedcentral.nih.gov.

WebMD. "Heart Disease Guide: Overview and Facts." www.webmd.com/heart disease/guide/heart-disease-overview-facts.

CHAPTER 1 — THE 10 BEST QUESTIONS ABOUT YOUR HEART ATTACK

Mayo Clinic. "Ejection Fraction: What Does It Measure?" www.mayoclinic.com/print/ejection-fraction/AN00360/METHOD=print.

MedicineNet. "Heart Attack." www.medicinenet.com/heart_attack/article.htm.

MedlinePlus. "Heart Attack." www.nlm.nih.gov/medlineplus/heartattack.html.

"Modern Treatment for Heart Attacks." *Circulation.* http://circ.ahajournals.org/cgi/content/full/114/20/e578.

National Heart Lung and Blood Institute. "What Is a Heart Attack?" www.nhlbi.nih.gov/health/dci/Diseases/HeartAttack/HeartAttack_WhatIs.html.

Rimmerman, Curtis. *Heart Attack.* Cleveland, OH: Cleveland Clinic Press, 2006.

Turner, Glenn O. *Recognizing and Surviving Heart Attacks and Strokes: Lifesaving Advice You Need Now.* Columbia, MO: University of Missouri Press, 2008.

CHAPTER 2 — THE 10 BEST QUESTIONS ABOUT YOUR HEART DISEASE

American Heart Association. "Heart Disease and Stroke Statistics." www.americanheart.org/downloadable/heart/1140534985281Statsupdate06book.pdf.

American Heart Association. "Tips for Talking to Healthcare Professionals." www.americanheart.org/presenter.jhtml?identifier=113.

British Heart Foundation. "Cardiovascular Disease." www.bhf.org.uk/living_with_heart_conditions/understanding_your_conditions/types_of_heart_conditions/coronary_heart_disease.aspx.

British Heart Foundation. "Our Most Popular BHF Publications." www.bhf.org.uk/living_with_heart_conditions/top_bhf_publications.aspx.

U.S. Department of Health and Human Services. National Institutes of Health. "Framingham Heart Study." www.nhlbi.nih.gov/about/framingham.

World Health Organization. "Cardiovascular Diseases." www.who.int/mediacentre/factsheets/fs317/en/index.html.

CHAPTER 3 — THE 10 BEST QUESTIONS TO GET RELIABLE REFERRALS FOR THE BEST DOCTORS AND SURGEONS

American Medical Association, "AMA ePhysician Profiles." www.ama-assn.org/ama/pub/category/2672.html.

Boston Central. "Doctor Referrals." www.bostoncentral.com/healthcare/doctor_ref.php.

Consumers' Checkbook. "Top Doctors." www.checkbook.org/doctors/pageone.cfm. (Subscription required.)

Gawande, Atul. *Better: A Surgeon's Notes on Performance.* New York: Henry Holt, 2007.

MedicineNet. "How to Choose a Doctor." www.medicinenet.com/script/main/art .asp?articlekey=47649.

Timmermans, Stefan, and Marc Berg. *The Gold Standard: The Challenge of Evidence-Based Medicine.* Philadelphia: Temple University Press, 2003.

CHAPTER 4 — THE 10 BEST QUESTIONS TO FIND A TOP CARDIOLOGIST OR CARDIAC SURGEON

American Board of Medical Specialties. "Bedside Manner, Board Certification Matter: Survey Reveals Top Qualities for Consumers Choosing a Doctor." www.abms.org/News_and_Events/Media_Newsroom/Releases/release_ ABMS_Consumer_Survey.aspx.

American Board of Medical Specialties. "How to Be a Smart Patient." www.abms .org/Who_We_Help/Consumers/educate.aspx.

American College of Surgeons. "Membership Database." http://web3.facs.org/acs dir/default_public.cfm.

Federation of State Medical Boards. "Welcome to DocInfo." www.docinfo.org.

National Institute on Aging. "Choosing a Doctor." www.nia.nih.gov/HealthInfor mation/Publications/choosing.htm.

National Medical Association. "Physician Locator." (Database of African-American physicians.) http://locator.fough3.com.

WebMD. "WebMD Physician Directory." http://doctor.webmd.com/physician_ finder/home.aspx?sponsor=core.

CHAPTER 5 — THE 10 BEST QUESTIONS FOR UNDERSTANDING DIAGNOSTIC TESTS AND CARDIAC PROCEDURES

American Heart Association. "Understanding Heart Failure." www.american heart.org/presenter.jhtml?identifier=1593.

American Heart Association. "What Is a Stress Test?" www.americanheart.org/ downloadable/heart/119620079524944%20WhatIsaStressTest%209_07 .pdf.

Cleveland Clinic Foundation. "Common Laboratory Tests." http://my.cleveland clinic.org/heart/services/tests/labtests/default.aspx.

Lab Tests Online. "Heart Disease: Tests." www.labtestsonline.org/understanding/ conditions/heart-4.html.

MedlinePlus. "Heart Disease: Diagnosis/Symptoms." www.nlm.nih.gov/medline
plus/heartdiseases.html#cat5.

National Heart Lung and Blood Institute. "Coronary Angiography: Key Points."
www.nhlbi.nih.gov/health/dci/Diseases/ca/ca_keypoints.html.

Texas Heart Institute. "Diagnostic Tests and Procedures." www.texasheartinstitute
.org/HIC/Topics/Diag.

CHAPTER 6 — THE 10 BEST QUESTIONS TO ASK WHEN GETTING A SECOND OPINION

Consumers' Checkbook. "Medical Advice— Is Your Doctor Measuring Up?" www
.checkbook.org. (Subscription required.)

Miller, Jim. "Savvy Senior: Second Opinion Can Buy Peace of Mind." *Charleston
Gazette.* May 10, 2004, p. 2D.

Thaler, Richard H., and Cass R. Sunstein. *Nudge: Improving Decisions About Health,
Wealth, and Happiness.* Caravan Books, 2008.

"When and How to Challenge Your Doctor." *U.S. News and World Report.* May 10,
1993, p. 62.

CHAPTER 7 — THE 10 BEST QUESTIONS ABOUT MANAGING YOUR RISK FACTORS FOR HEART DISEASE

American Diabetes Association. "All About Diabetes." www.diabetes.org/about
diabetes.jsp.

American Heart Association. "Cholesterol." www.americanheart.org/presenter
.jhtml?identifier=1516.

American Heart Association. "Lifestyle and Risk Reduction." www.american
heart.org/presenter.jhtml?identifier=3004354#Smoking.

American Lung Association. "Quit Smoking." www.lungusa.org/site/pp
.asp?c=dvLUK9O0E&b=33484.

British Heart Foundation. "Family History." www.bhf.org.uk/keeping_your_
heart_healthy/preventing_heart_disease/family_history.aspx.

Centers for Disease Control and Prevention. "Defining Overweight and Obesity."
www.cdc.gov/nccdphp/dnpa/obesity/defining.htm.

MedlinePlus. "Cholesterol." www.nlm.nih.gov/medlineplus/cholesterol.html.

National Heart Lung and Blood Institute. "What Is High Blood Pressure?" www
.nhlbi.nih.gov/health/dci/Diseases/Hbp/HBP_WhatIs.html.

Wikipedia. "Physical Exercise." http://en.wikipedia.org/wiki/Exercise.

World Heart Federation. "Cardiovascular Disease Risk Factors." www.world-heart
-federation.org/cardiovascular-health/cardiovascular-disease-risk-factors.

CHAPTER 8 — THE 10 BEST QUESTIONS FOR WOMEN ABOUT HEART HEALTH

Berra, Kathleen, et al. *Heart Attack!: Advice for Patients by Patients.* New Haven, CT: Yale University Press, 2001.

Cleveland Clinic. "Women's Heart: Menopause Increases the Risk of Heart Attack and Stroke." http://my.clevelandclinic.org/newsletters/heart/2007summer /menopause.aspx.

Kastan, Kathy. *From the Heart: A Woman's Guide to Living Well with Heart Disease.* New York: Da Capo Lifelong Books, 2007.

National Heart Lung and Blood Institute. "Healthy Heart Handbook for Women." www.nhlbi.nih.gov/health/public/heart/other/hhw/index.htm.

National Heart Lung and Blood Institute. "Heart Truth: A National Awareness Campaign for Women About Heart Disease." www.hearttruth.gov.

Serure, Pamela. *Take It to Heart: The Real Deal On Women and Heart Disease.* New York: Broadway, 2006.

CHAPTER 9 — THE 10 BEST QUESTIONS TO ASK ABOUT HEART MEDICATIONS

American Heart Association. "What Are Anticoagulants and Antiplatelet Agents?" www.americanheart.org/downloadable/heart/1196965757160Anti coagandAntiplat.pdf.

American Pharmacists Association. "Pharmacy and You." www.pharmacyandyou .org.

Food and Drug Administration. "Patient Information Fact Sheets." www.fda.gov/ cder/drug/infopage/antipsychotics/default.htm.

HeartHelp. "Heart Medications." www.hearthelp.com/heartfailure/medications .html.

Medicare. "Medicare Prescription Drug Plan Finder." www.medicare.gov.

MedlinePlus. "Drugs, Supplements, and Herbal Information." (Database search- able by drug name.) www.nlm.nih.gov/medlineplus/druginformation.html.

PhRMA. "Publications." www.phrma.org/publications.com/conditions/heart/ heart-attack/recovery-guide/medications.

U.S. Pharmacopeia. "USP's Drug Error Finder." www.usp.org/hqi/similarProd ucts/drugErrorFinderTool.html.

CHAPTER 10 — THE 10 BEST QUESTIONS ABOUT HEART SURGERY

American College of Surgeons. "When You Need an Operation: About Carotid Endarterectomy." www.facs.org/public_info/operation/brochures/carotid.pdf.

American Heart Association. "How Can I Recover from Heart Surgery?" www
.americanheart.org/downloadable/heart/1196355902375RecoverHeartSurgery
.pdf.

American Heart Association. "Minimally Invasive Heart Surgery." www.ameri
canheart.org/presenter.jhtml?identifier=4702.

American Heart Association. "What Is Coronary Bypass Surgery?" www.ameri
canheart.org/downloadable/heart/119626671501548%20WhatIsCornry
BypsSrgry_9-07.pdf.

National Heart Lung and Blood Institute. "Facts About Angioplasty." www.nhlbi
.nih.gov/health/dci/Diseases/Angioplasty/Angioplasty_WhatIs.html.

Society of Thoracic Surgeons. "What to Expect After Heart Surgery." www.sts.org/
sections/patientinformation/adultcardiacsurgery/heartsurgery.

"Too Much Treatment?" *Consumer Reports.* July 2008, pp. 40–44.

CHAPTER 11—THE 10 BEST QUESTIONS FOR CHOOSING A HOSPITAL

American Hospital Association. "Consumer Health Care Information." www.aha
.org/aha_app/resource-center/links/consumer-links.jsp.

American Nurses Association. "Patient Safety & Quality." www.nursingworld
.org/MainMenuCategories/ThePracticeofProfessionalNursing/PatientSafety
Quality.aspx.

BBC.co.uk. "Talking to Your Doctor—In the Hospital: Inpatient Checklist."
www.bbc.co.uk/health/talking_to_your_doctor/hospital_checklist.shtml.

Buck, Jari Holland. *Hospital Stay Handbook: A Guide to Becoming a Patient Advocate
for Your Loved Ones.* St. Paul, MN: Llewellyn Publications, 2007.

National Patient Safety Foundation. "Safety as You Go from Hospital to Home."
www.npsf.org/download/SafetyAsYouGo.pdf.

U.S. Department of Health and Human Services. "20 Tips to Help Prevent Medi
cal Errors: Patient Fact Sheet." www.ahrq.gov/consumer/20tips.htm.

USNews.Com. "Directory of America's Hospitals: Guarding Against Mistakes."
www.usnews.com/usnews/health/hospitals/articles/mistakes.htm.

Wikipedia. "Medical Errors." http://en.wikipedia.org/wiki/Medical_errors.

CHAPTER 12—THE 10 BEST QUESTIONS ABOUT CARDIAC REHABILITATION

British Heart Foundation. "Cardiac Rehabilitation: Health Information Series
Number 23." www.bhf.org.uk/publications.aspx?sPage=3.

Canadian Cardiac Rehabilitation Foundation. "Cardiac Rehabilitation Centres
Across Canada." www.cardiacrehabilitation.ca/rehab_centres.php.

252 · Bibliography

"Heart Disease: New Heart Disease Study Findings Have Been Reported by Researchers at Mayo Clinic." *Heart Disease Weekly.* July 12, 2008, p. 50.

O'Neill, John. Rehabilitation and Heart Disease." *New York Times.* September 7, 2004, p. F6.

Quest Diagnostics. "Cardiac Rehabilitation." www.questdiagnostics.com/kbase/topic/special/hw229962/sec6.htm.

Southard, Douglas R., et al. "Core Competencies for Cardiac Rehabilitation Professionals." *Journal of Cardiopulmonary Rehabilitation.* Vol. 14, Number 2, March 20, 1994. www.aacvpr.org/members/statements/CoreCompCardiac.pdf.

CHAPTER 13—THE 10 BEST QUESTIONS FOR CHOOSING ALTERNATIVE TREATMENTS FOR HEART DISEASE

American Board of Medical Specialties. "Online Physician Ratings: Proceed with Caution." www.abms.org/News_and_Events/Media_Newsroom/Releases/release_PhysiciansRatings_06_11_08.aspx.

Better Business Bureau. "For Consumers." http://us.bbb.org/WWWRoot/SitePage.aspx?site=113&id=b81f1c7b-c315-4f43-8d92-a44a2248ec44.

Consumer Healthcare Products Association. "Dietary Supplements Are Regulated Products." www.chpa-info.org/ChpaPortal/issues/DSHEA/Dietarysupplements.htm.

Federal Citizen Information Center. "State, County, and City Government Consumer Protection Offices." www.consumeraction.gov/state.shtml.

Federal Trade Commission. "Virtual 'Treatments' Can Be Real-World Deceptions." www.ftc.gov/bcp/conline/pubs/alerts/mrclalrt.shtm.

Food and Drug Administration. "Buying Prescription Medicine Online: A Consumer Safety Guide." www.fda.gov/cder/consumerinfo/buyOnlineGuide_text.htm.

Health on the Net Foundation. "HONcode Site Evaluation Form." www.hon.ch/HONcode/HONcode_check.html.

MedlinePlus. "MedlinePlus Guide to Healthy Web Surfing." www.nlm.nih.gov/medlineplus/healthywebsurfing.html.

National Center for Complementary and Alternative Medicine. "Herbal Supplements: Consider Safety, Too." www.nccam.nih.gov/health/supplement-safety.

National Consumer's League. "Home Page." www.nclnet.org/fraud.

URAC. "Consumer Resource Center." www.urac.org/consumers/resources.

Weil, Andrew. *Healthy Aging: A Lifelong Guide to Your Physical and Spiritual Well-Being.* New York: Knopf, 2005.

Weil, Andrew. *Natural Health, Natural Medicine: The Complete Guide to Wellness and Self-Care for Optimum Health,* rev. ed. Boston: Houghton Mifflin, 2004.

CHAPTER 14—THE 10 BEST QUESTIONS TO TAME YOUR STRESS

About.com. "Chronic Job Stress Is a Risk Factor for Heart Disease." http://stress.about.com/od/stresshealth/a/jobstress.htm.

American Psychological Association. "Find a Psychologist." http://locator.apa.org.

Canadian Centre for Occupational Health and Safety. Workplace Stress: General." www.ccohs.org/ohsanswers/psychosocial/stress.html.

Maxon, Rebecca. "Stress in the Workplace: A Costly Epidemic." Fairleigh Dickinson University. www.fdu.edu/newspubs/magazine/99su/stress.html.

Mayo Clinic. "Job Burnout: Know the Signs and Symptoms." www.mayoclinic.com/health/burnout/WL00062.

MedicineNet. "Heart Disease: Stress and Heart Disease." www.medicinenet.com/stress_and_heart_disease/article.htm.

WebMD. "Heart Disease: Stress and Heart Disease." www.webmd.com/heart-disease/stress-heart-attack-risk.

CHAPTER 15—THE 10 BEST QUESTIONS TO LOSE WEIGHT AND EAT HEALTHY

American Council on Exercise. "Fit Facts: Weight." www.acefitness.org/fitfacts/default.aspx#Choosing%20Fitness%20Trainers%20and%20Instructors.

Heart Foundation. "Healthy Weight." www.heartfoundation.org.au/Healthy_Living/Healthy_Weight.htm.

McGee, Harold. *On Food and Cooking: The Science and Lore of the Kitchen.* New York: Scribner, 2004.

Ornish, Dean. *Dr. Dean Ornish's Program for Reversing Heart Disease: The Only System Scientifically Proven to Reverse Heart Disease Without Drugs or Surgery.* New York: Ballantine Books, 2008.

Sinatra, Stephen, and James C. Roberts. *Reverse Heart Disease Now: Stop Deadly Cardiovascular Plaque Before It's Too Late.* New York: John Wiley & Sons, 2007.

Willett, Walter C., and P.J. Skerrett. *Eat, Drink, and Be Healthy: The Harvard Medical School Guide to Healthy Eating.* New York: Free Press, 2005.

CHAPTER 16 — THE 10 BEST QUESTIONS TO FIND A GREAT GYM OR FITNESS CLUB

American College of Sports Medicine. "Selecting and Effectively Using a Health/ Fitness Facility." www.acsm.org/AM/Template.cfm?Section=Brochures2& Template=/CM/ContentDisplay.cfm&ContentID=8100.

American Council on Exercise. "Fit Facts: Exercising with Health Challenges." www.acefitness.org/fitfacts/default.aspx#Choosing%20Fitness%20Train ers%20and%20Instructors.

American Council on Exercise. "The Right Exercise Program for You Starts Here." www.acefitness.org/fitfacts/fitfacts_display.aspx?itemid=50.

President's Council on Physical Fitness and Sports. "Physical Activity Facts." www.fitness.gov/resources/facts/index.html.

Quest Diagnostics. "Exercise Tips If You Have a Pacemaker or ICD." www.quest diagnostics.com/kbase/frame/ty642/ty6423abc/frame.htm.

Sonnemaker, Bill. "Current Articles." www.fitnesscatalyst.com/Current-Articles .html.

CHAPTER 17 — THE 10 BEST QUESTIONS TO HIRE A TOP PERSONAL TRAINER

About.com. "10 Reasons to Fire Your Personal Trainer." http://exercise.about .com/od/personaltraining/tp/firepersonaltra.htm.

About.com. "Choosing a Personal Trainer: Warning Flags." http://exercise.about .com/cs/forprofessionals/a/choosetrainer_2.htm.

American Council on Exercise. "Reap the Rewards of Personal Training." www .acefitness.org/fitfacts/fitfacts_display.aspx?itemid=93.

Body Building for You. "How to Choose a Certified Personal Trainer to Meet Your Needs." www.bodybuildingforyou.com/articles-submit/ghf/choose-personal -trainer.htm.

Quackwatch. "How to Choose a Personal Trainer." www.quackwatch.org/04 ConsumerEducation/trainer.html.

CHAPTER 18 — THE 10 BEST QUESTIONS TO BREAK NICOTINE'S GRIP

American Heart Association. "Personal Support and Local Resources to Help You Quit Smoking." www.americanheart.org/presenter.jhtml?identifier=3049334.

American Heart Association. "Quitting Smoking." www.americanheart.org/pre senter.jhtml?identifier=3048036.

American Lung Association. "Smoking 101 Fact Sheet." www.lungusa.org/site/ c.dvLUK9O0E/b.39853/k.5D05/Smoking_101_Fact_Sheet.htm.

Mayo Clinic. "Quit Smoking." www.mayoclinic.com/health/quit-smoking/QS99999.

Medline Plus. "Local Smoking Cessation Resources." www.nlm.nih.gov/medline plus/golocal/topicmap_1359.html.

National Cancer Institute. "Learn How to Quit Smoking: Print Resources." www .smokefree.gov/resources.html.

National Institutes of Health. "Clinical Trials on Smoking Cessation." http://clin icaltrials.gov/search/open/condition=%22Smoking+Cessation%22.

CHAPTER 19—THE 10 BEST QUESTIONS TO ASSESS YOUR DRINKING HABITS

Alcoholics Anonymous. "Alcoholism and Alcoholics." www.alcoholics-anony mous.org/en_is_aa_for you.cfm?PageID=13&SubPage=77.

American Medical Association. "AMA Policies on Alcohol." www.ama-assn.org/ ama/pub/category/3342.html.

Betty Ford Clinic. "Do You Have a Problem with Alcohol or Other Drugs?" www .bettyfordcenter.org/admissions/index.php?ql=problem.

Hanson, David J. *Preventing Alcohol Abuse: Alcohol, Culture, and Control.* Westport, CT: Praeger Publishers, 1995.

Johns Hopkins University. "Alcohol and Heart Attacks—Does a Drink a Day Lower Your Risk?" www.johnshopkinshealthalerts.com/reports/heart_health /265-1.html?CMP=OTC-RSS.

National Institute on Alcohol Abuse and Alcoholism. "Tips for Cutting Down Drinking." http://pubs.niaaa.nih.gov/publications/Tips/tips.pdf.

Wikipedia. "Paddington Alcohol Test." http://en.wikipedia.org/wiki/Padding ton_Alcohol_Test.

CHAPTER 20—THE 10 BEST QUESTIONS FOR EMOTIONAL HEALTH FOR HEART PATIENTS

Budnick, Herbert N. *Heart to Heart: A Guide to the Psychological Aspects of Heart Disease.* Albuquerque, NM: Health Press NA Inc., 2007.

Cleveland Clinic. Women's Heart: Stay Calm—Your Heart Will Thank You." http://my.clevelandclinic.org/newsletters/heart/2007summer/staycalm.aspx.

Depression.com. "Web Resources." www.depression.com/web_resources.html.

Laman, Kirk. *How to Heal Your Broken Heart: A Cardiologist's Secrets for Physical, Emotional, and Spiritual Health.* Charleston, SC: Advantage Media Group, 2006.

Lerner, Harriet. *The Dance of Anger: A Woman's Guide to Changing the Patterns of Intimate Relationships.* New York: Harper Paperbacks, 2005.

Lotsa Helping Hands. "How It Works." www.lotsahelpinghands.com/ltc/how.

CHAPTER 21 — THE 10 BEST QUESTIONS WHEN TALKING WITH YOUR PARTNER AFTER A HEART ATTACK

American Association for Marriage and Family Therapy. "Search for a Marriage and Family Therapist Near You." www.therapistlocator.net.

American Heart Association. "Caregiver's Guide." www.americanheart.org/pre senter.jhtml?identifier=1412.

Levin, Aaron. Center for the Advancement of Health. "Spouses' Negative Emotions Can Alter Heart Attack Recovery." September 10, 2004. www.cfah.org/hbns/news/heartattack09-10-04.cfm.

Moore, Thomas. *Soul Mates*. New York: Harper Perennial, 1994.

National Alliance for Caregiving. "Welcome!" www.caregiving.org.

National Family Caregivers Association. "Caregiving Resources." www.nfcacares .org/caregiving_resources.

CHAPTER 22 — THE 10 BEST QUESTIONS FOR SEXUAL HEALTH AND INTIMACY AFTER A HEART ATTACK

Chapunoff, Eduardo. *Sex and the Cardiac Patient: A Practical Guide*. Bendy Books, 1991.

Cole, Harriette, and John Pinderhughes. *Coming Together: Celebrations for African-American Families*. New York: Jump in the Sun Publishers, 2003.

Lerner, Harriet. *The Dance of Intimacy*. New York: Harper Paperbacks, 2005.

Reinisch, June M., and Ruth Beasley. *The Kinsey Institute New Report on Sex: What You Must Know to Be Sexually Literate*. New York: St. Martin's Press, 1990.

Rose, Tricia. *Longing to Tell: Black Women Talk About Sexuality and Intimacy*. New York: Picador, 2004.

CHAPTER 23 — THE 10 BEST QUESTIONS BEFORE JOINING A SUPPORT GROUP

CardioSmart. "Make Connections." www.cardiosmart.org/MakeConnections.

Kurtz, Linda. *Self-Help and Support Groups: A Handbook for Practitioners*. Thousand Oaks, CA: Sage Publications, 1997.

National Self-Help Clearinghouse. "What Is Self-Help and How Does It Work?" www.selfhelpweb.org/what.html#what.

Schiff, Harriet Sarnoff. *The Support Group Manual: A Session-by-Session Guide*. New York: Penguin Books, 1996.

Schwarz, Roger. *The Skilled Facilitator*, 2nd ed. San Francisco: Jossey-Bass, 2002.

Warnock, Sheila. *Share the Care: How to Organize a Group to Care for Someone Who Is Seriously Ill.* New York: Fireside, 2004.

Well Spouse Foundation. "Support Groups by State." www.wellspouse.org/index .php?option=com_contxtd&Itemid=50.

CHAPTER 24—THE 10 BEST QUESTIONS FOR A HEART PATIENT'S FINANCIAL HEALTH

American Bar Association. "Commission on Law and Aging." www.abanet.org/ aging.

American Bar Association. "Consumers' Guide to Legal Help." www.abanet.org/ legalservices/findlegalhelp/home.cfm.

American Heart Association. "Financial Concerns." www.americanheart.org/pre senter.jhtml?identifier=335.

Burns, Sharon, and Raymond Forgue. *How to Care for Your Parents' Money While Caring for Your Parents.* New York: McGraw-Hill, 2003.

Heart Support of America. "Patient Services." (Provides financial assistance.) www .heartsupportofamerica.org/patient_services.shtml.

National Academy of Elder Law Attorneys. "Locate an Elder Law Attorney." http:// naela.ebiz.uapps.net/solutionsite/Default.aspx?tabid=148.

National Foundation for Credit Counseling. "Consumer Debt Advice." www .debtadvice.org.

National Institute on Aging. "Getting Your Affairs in Order." www.nia.nih.gov/ HealthInformation/Publications/affairs.htm.

Partnership for Prescription Assistance. (Searchable database for patient and caregiver programs.) www.pparx.org.

CHAPTER 25—THE 10 WORST QUESTIONS TO ASK A HEART PATIENT

Birnbach, Lisa, and Patricia Marx. *1,003 Great Things About Getting Older.* Kansas City, MO: Andrews McMeel Publishing, 1997.

Metcalf, C. W., and Roma Felible. *Lighten Up: Survival Skills for People Under Pressure.* New York: Perseus Books, 1992.

Sherman, James R. *The Magic of Humor in Caregiving.* Golden Valley, MN: Pathway Books, 1995.

CHAPTER 26 — THE 10 BEST QUESTIONS FOR SPIRITUAL HEALTH
FOR HEART PATIENTS

Association of Professional Chaplains. "Healing Spirit." (Newsletter.) www.pro fessionalchaplains.org/index.aspx?id=678.

Duke University: Center for Spirituality, Theology, and Health. "Research and Publications." www.dukespiritualityandhealth.org/publications.

Institute for the Study of Health and Illness. "Finding Meaning in Medicine." www.meaninginmedicine.org/home.html.

Spirituality & Health. "Articles." www.spirituality-health.com/spirit/content /articles.

Tzu, Lao. Tao Te Ching: A New English Version. New York: Harper, 2006.

University of Florida Center for Spirituality and Health. "Bibliographies." www .spiritualityandhealth.ufl.edu/bibliographies.

Warren, Rick. The Purpose-Driven Life: What on Earth Am I Here For? Grand Rapids, MI: Zondervan Press, 2002.

Young, Caroline, and Cyndie Koopsen. Spirituality, Health and Healing. Sudbury, MA: Jones and Barlett Publishers, 2005.

Meet the Experts

The author interviewed each of the following experts for this book.

Rebecca Allison, MD, FACC, FACP, is an experienced cardiologist in Phoenix, Arizona, the president-elect for the Gay and Lesbian Medical Association, and chair of the American Medical Association's advisory committee on gay and lesbian issues. Dr. Allison has been chosen by peers as one of *Phoenix* magazine's "Top Doctors" in Phoenix for several years.

Stephen Barrett, MD, a retired psychiatrist in Allentown, Pennsylvania, is an author, editor, and consumer advocate best known for his popular Web site, Quackwatch. Quackwatch, Inc., is a nonprofit organization whose mission is to "combat health-related frauds, myths, fads, fallacies, and misconduct" while providing "quackery-related information that is difficult or impossible to get elsewhere." His Web site is www.quackwatch.org.

Hamilton Beazley, PhD, is the scholar-in-residence at St. Edward's University in Austin, Texas, and the author of *No Regrets: A Ten-Step Program for Living in the Present and Leaving the Past Behind.* Dr. Beazley has been interviewed on *Oprah,* NBC, CNN, and many other television and radio shows and networks. The Web site is www.stedwards.edu.

Herbert Benson, MD, is a world-renowned pioneer in mind–body medicine, director emeritus of the Benson-Henry Institute for Mind Body Medicine at Massachusetts General Hospital, and a former Harvard University professor. Dr. Benson has written more than one hundred eighty scientific publications and eleven books, including the best-seller *The Relaxation Response* (1975). His institute's Web site is www.mbmi.org and his Wikipedia entry is at http://en.wikipedia.org/wiki/Herbert_Benson.

Norman Berk is a certified financial planner, CPA, personal financial specialist, and JD. He founded Professional Asset Strategies, LLC, a fee-only financial firm in Birmingham, Alabama. Both he and his wife are cancer survivors and activists. His Web site is http://proassetsllc.com.

Kathy Berra, MSN, NP-C, FAAN, is the clinical director of the Stanford Heart Network for online cardiovascular health assessment and health education. She is also a nurse practitioner at Cardiovascular Medicine and Coronary Interventions and coauthor of an award-winning book. Ms. Berra has over thirty-five years in cardiac care and is the past president of the American Association of Cardiovascular and Pulmonary Rehabilitation and the Preventive Cardiovascular Nurses Association. The Web site is www.stanford.edu.

Lorraine Biros, LCPC, is the director for client services and a licensed clinical professional counselor at the Mautner Project: The National Lesbian Health Organization in Washington, D.C. Ms. Biros has more than twenty-eight years of counseling experience in the lesbian and gay community. The organization's Web site is www.mautnerproject.org.

Jessica Black, ND, is a naturopathic physician in private practice in McMinnville, Oregon, and author of the book *The Anti-Inflammation Diet and Recipe Book.* Dr. Black specializes in complementary therapies, pediatrics, and women's medicine in-

cluding natural hormone balancing. Her Web site is www.afami
lyhealingcenter.com.

William Blatt, MPH is the manager of tobacco control programs at
the American Lung Association National Headquarters and oversees
all of the association's tobacco prevention and cessation programs.
He was responsible for the 2007 edition of the adult cessation program Freedom From Smoking® and is supervising the creation of
the 2009 edition of the youth cessation program, Not On Tobacco®.
The American Lung Association's Web site is www.lungusa.org.

Peter Block has an international reputation as a management con-
sultant and as the author of best-selling books, including *Flawless
Consulting: A Guide to Getting Your Expertise Used* and *The Answer to
How Is Yes,* a book that examines the underlying assumptions about
asking questions. His newest book is *Community: The Structure of
Belonging,* and his Web site is www.peterblock.com.

Alfred Bove, MD, PhD, FACC, is the 2008–2009 president of
the American College of Cardiology, and is the former chief of cardiology and emeritus professor of medicine at Temple University
Medical Center. He served as chief editor of Cardiosource.com and
has published more than two hundred fifty original research papers
and books on coronary disease and environmental medicine during
his forty years in medicine. The Web sites are www.temple.edu,
www.cardiosource.com, www.acc.org, and www.scubamed.com.

Barbara (Bobbi) P. Clarke, PhD, RD, is a professor, health specialist, and codirector for the University of Tennessee's Center for
Community Health Literacy. She has more than thirty years of experience in public health education and community development.
Dr. Clarke leads a community health program delivered through-

out Tennessee to improve health literacy and to help people make health decisions. The program's Web site is http://fcs.tennessee .edu/healthsafety/phealth.htm.

Harriette Cole is a professional life coach, has authored several books, and reaches a broad multiethnic audience with her nationally syndicated advice column, "Sense and Sensitivity." Ms. Cole is currently the creative director of *Ebony* magazine, heads Harriette Cole Productions, and coaches recording artists including notable musicians such as JoJo, Alicia Keys, and Mary J. Blige. Her Web site is www.harriettecole.com and her Wikipedia entry is at http:// en.wikipedia.org/wiki/Harriette_Cole.

Caldwell B. Esselstyn, Jr., MD, is a clinician and the author of the best-selling book *Prevent and Reverse Heart Disease.* Since 1968 he has been associated with the Cleveland Heart Clinic, including as staff president. Dr. Esselstyn was awarded the Benjamin Spock Award for Compassion in Medicine, has published over one hundred fifty scientific papers, and was chosen as one of the 1994–1995 "Best Doctors in America." His Web site is www.heartattackproof.com.

Caela Farren, PhD, founder and CEO of MasteryWorks, Inc., in Falls Church, Virginia, has over thirty years of experience as an international consultant, entrepreneur, and educator. Dr. Farren has also authored several popular books including *Who's Running Your Career* and *Designing Career Development Systems,* as well as numerous journal articles. She survived a heart attack in 2004. Her Web site is www.masteryworks.com.

Betty Ferrell, RN, PhD, FAAN, is a clinician and research scientist in pain management at City of Hope National Medical Center in Duarte, California. She has been in nursing for more than thirty years and focuses on spirituality issues, quality of life, and palliative care. Dr. Ferrell is a Fellow of the American Academy of Nursing and has authored over two hundred seventy publications including five books on pain management and nursing care. The Web site is www.cityofhope.org/Pages/default.aspx.

Edwin B. Fisher, PhD, is a professor in the Department of Health Behavior and Health Education in the School of Public Health at the University of North Carolina at Chapel Hill. He is also global director of the American Academy of Family Physicians Foundation's project, *Peers for Progress,* an international program to promote peer support for diabetes management. For more than twenty-five years, Dr. Fisher has been a leading expert, researcher, and international contributor to smoking cessation efforts. He is widely published, including the books 7 *Steps to a Smoke Free Life* (1998) and *How to Quit Smoking Without Gaining Weight* (2004).

Daniel Forman, MD, is an assistant professor of medicine at the Harvard Medical School and the director of the Exercise Testing Laboratory and Cardiac Rehabilitation at the Brigham and Women's Hospital in Boston. He is also a staff physician at the Geriatric Research, Education and Clinical Care Center for the Veterans Administration. Dr. Forman has done extensive research on cardiovascular disease and preventive lifestyle modifications.

Rachael Freed, MSW, LMFT, has practiced psychotherapy for thirty years, founded Women's Legacies, and authored *Heartmates: A Guide for the Spouse and Family of the Heart Patient,* 3rd edition (2002), *The Heartmates Journal: A Companion for Partners of People with Serious Illness* (2002), and *Women's Lives, Women's Legacies* (2003). Ms. Freed trains professionals, facilitates legacy writing, and is a senior fellow at the University of Minnesota's Center for Spirituality and Healing. Her Web sites are www.Heartmates.com and www.womenslegacies.com.

Timothy J. Gardner, MD, is the current national president of the American Heart Association, serving as its chief volunteer science and medical officer. Dr. Gardner is also the medical director of the Center for Heart & Vascular Health at the Christiana Care Health System in Newark, Delaware. A nationally noted heart surgeon and cardiovascular medicine leader, Dr. Gardner has authored nearly two hundred scientific papers. The Web sites are www.american heart.org and www.christiancare.org.

Mark Gorkin, MSW, LICSW, is a licensed clinical social worker who calls himself "The Stress Doc." Mr. Gorkin is a motivational speaker, humorist, organizational consultant, and the author of two books on stress management. His Web site is www.stressdoc.com.

John Gray, PhD, is the world's number one–selling relationship author. An international gender and relationship expert, his *New York Times* best-selling *Men Are from Mars, Women Are from Venus* books have sold more than thirty million copies worldwide. His principles have helped millions of couples. Dr. Gray's latest book, *Why Mars and Venus Collide,* is available at www.marsvenus.com/collide and his Wikipedia entry is at http://en.wikipedia.org/wiki/John_Gray_(U.S._author).

Mimi Guarneri, MD, FACC, is the medical director of the Scripps Center for Integrative Medicine in La Jolla, California. She co-founded the center in 1999 to address patients' emotional, spiritual, and physical needs. Dr. Guarneri has authored numerous professional articles and the book *The Heart Speaks: A Cardiologist Reveals the Secret Language of Healing.* The Web site is www.scripps

.org/locations/scripps-clinic/services/integrative-medicine_integra
tive-medicine.

Larry F. Hamm, PhD, FAACVPR, FACSM, is the current president of the American Association of Cardiovascular and Pulmonary
Rehabilitation and director of the Clinical Exercise Physiology Program at The George Washington University Medical Center in
Washington, D.C. He has more than thirty years in cardiac rehabilitation, a PhD in exercise physiology, and is certified by the
American College of Sports Medicine as a program director for exercise programs. The Web site is www.aacvpr.org.

David J. Hanson, PhD, is a professor emeritus of sociology at the
State University of New York at Potsdam and an international expert
on alcohol consumption. Dr. Hanson has written more than three
hundred papers and books, studied alcohol consumption for more
than forty years, and appeared on dozens of national television and
radio programs. His Web site is www.alcoholinformation.org and his
Wikipedia entry is http://en.wikipedia.org/wiki/David_J._Hanson.

Sharonne N. Hayes, MD, FACC, is the director of the Mayo Clinic
Women's Heart Clinic in Rochester, Minnesota, and an associate
professor of medicine. She developed this clinic to meet the unique
needs of women with heart disease and with cardiovascular risk,
improve patient satisfaction, and offer preventive cardiology and
research. Dr. Hayes is a nationally recognized speaker on women's
cardiovascular health, including television appearances on *Charlie
Rose* and the *Today* show. The Web site is www.mayoclinic.org.

Julie R. Heiman, PhD, is the director of the famous Kinsey Institute for Research in Sex, Gender and Reproduction at Indiana University in Bloomington, Indiana. For more than sixty years the

Kinsey Institute has been the worldwide pioneer and leader in studying human sexuality, gender, and reproduction research. Dr. Heiman's research interests include sexual arousal and traumatic sexual experiences. The Web site is www.kinseyinstitute.org.

Peggy Jensen, RD, MBA, has more than twenty-five years as a registered dietitian, including work in New York City developing a "cardiac prudent diet" for her cardiac patients and their families. Ms. Jensen coordinated a nutritional educational program for the American Heart Association in New York on heart-healthy cooking, shopping, and dining out. Ms. Jensen currently owns a nutrition consulting business and teaches school in Virginia.

Sharon Jordan-Evans is the president of the Jordan Evans Group, a speaker, and a workplace consultant. She is also a certified coach and the coauthor of two best-selling books on workplace issues: *Love 'Em or Lose 'Em: Getting Good People to Stay* and *Love It, Don't Leave It: 26 Ways to Get What You Want at Work.* Her Web site is www.jeg.org.

Spencer B. King, III, MD, MACC, is the executive director of academic affairs and the interim president of the Saint Joseph's Heart and Vascular Institute in Atlanta, Georgia. Dr. King specializes in interventional cardiology and is professor emeritus (cardiology) at Emory University. He is the past president of the American College of Cardiology and has authored more than five hundred articles and ten books. The Web site is www.stjosephsatlanta.org/heart_and_vascular_institute.

Paul Kligfield, MD, is a professor of medicine at the Weill Medical College of Cornell University and medical director of the Cardiac Health Center in New York City. His popular book, *The*

Cardiac Recovery Handbook: The Complete Guide to Life After Heart Attack or Heart Surgery, covers all aspects of cardiac recovery. Dr. Kligfield graduated from Harvard Medical School. The Web site is www.med.cornell.edu.

Richard Koonce is president of Richard Koonce Productions, Inc., a human resources consulting and communications firm in Brookline, Massachusetts. Mr. Koonce is an experienced writer, consultant, facilitator, coach, and interviewer and has authored four business books. His Web site is www.richardkoonce.com.

C. Everett Koop, MD, was the U.S. surgeon general from 1982 to 1989. He is the recipient of numerous awards, including seventeen honorary doctorate degrees and the Presidential Medal of Freedom. Still going strong at ninety plus years old, Dr. Koop stays current with medical education and patient care issues. During his tenure as a high-profile surgeon general and throughout his long career, Dr. Koop has been an outspoken advocate for improving patient–physician communications. His Wikipedia biography is at http://en.wikipedia.org/wiki/C._Everett_Koop.

Dorothy Leeds, MA, is an internationally acclaimed bestselling author, trainer, keynoter, sales consultant, and expert in questioning skills. Known as the "Questioning Crusader," she has written twelve books including *The 7 Powers of Questions* (2000). Her media exposure includes NBC's *Today* show, ABC's *Good Morning America,* and *The New York Times.* Ms. Leeds also appears in Broadway shows. Her Web site is www.dorothyleeds.com.

Anna Maravelas, Licensed Psychologist, MA, is an international consultant specializing in stress and conflict in the workplace. She is the author of *How to Reduce Workplace Conflict and Stress* (2005) and the founder of TheraRising, Inc., in St. Paul, Minnesota. She teaches leaders to avoid the "Self-Defeating Habits of Otherwise Brilliant People: Pulling in Together When Things Fall Apart." Ms. Maravelas's work has appeared in *The New York Times, Forbes, O: The Oprah Magazine,* and *Harvard Management Update.* Her Web site is http://therarising.com.

Cicily Carson Maton is a certified financial planner and the founder of Aequus Wealth Management Resources, a Chicago-based financial planning and investment firm that specializes in advising people during major life transitions. She has appeared several times on the television show *Right on the Money.* Her Web site is www.aequus wealth.com.

Rear Admiral Kenneth P. Moritsugu, MD, MPH, retired in 2007 as the acting U.S. surgeon general in Washington, D.C. Admiral Moritsugu's forty years in public health service included many honors, such as his service as deputy surgeon general for nearly ten years. Admiral Moritsugu's Wikipedia biography is at http://en.wikipedia.org/wiki/Kenneth_P._Moritsugu.

Debbie Nigro is an award-winning radio personality, champion of women, author, speaker, and business executive based in New York. Ms. Nigro has interviewed hundreds of people for her radio shows, which are aired in four hundred fifty markets. She is also president of Out of the Box Deals, Inc., a public relations firm in New Rochelle. Her Web site is www.firstwivesworld.com.

Scott Peck, PhD, and **Shannon Peck,** of San Diego, California, cofounded TheLoveCenter, an educational organization dedicated to raising relationship and spiritual awareness, and have coauthored several books. Their Web site is www.thelovecenter.com.

Christina M. Puchalski, MD, directs the Institute for Spirituality and Health (GWish), is an associate professor of medicine at The George Washington University in Washington, D.C., and is a practicing physician. Dr. Puchalski is an internationally recognized pioneer in the integration of spirituality and health care and author of the book *A Time for Listening and Caring: Spirituality and the Care of the Chronically Ill and Dying.* The Web site is www.gwish.org.

Vicki Rackner, MD, is a board-certified surgeon who left the operating room to help patients, patients' families, and caregivers partner more effectively with their doctors through her company, Medical Bridges. She is also an author, speaker, and consultant, including coauthor of a *Chicken Soup for the Soul: Healthy Living Series* book and several patient self-help books. Her Web site is www.medicalbridges.com.

Samuel M. Schwartz, PhD, has survived two heart attacks and two bypass surgeries since 1977. Now retired and living in Chevy Chase, Maryland, Dr. Schwartz was formerly a senior manager at the National Institutes of Health, where he was responsible for conducting peer reviews of major biomedical grants.

Paul Schyve, MD, is senior vice president of The Joint Commission and has specialized in assessing hospital quality and patient care for more than twenty-two years. The organization's Web site is www.jointcommission.org.

Susan Sikora hosts a television talk show in San Francisco, California, called *Bay Area Focus with Susan Sikora* and has interviewed hundreds of political, entertainment, and health celebrities. Ms. Sikora is an Emmy winner who formerly hosted live talk shows for PBS, CBS, NBC, and ABC. The Web site is http://cwbayarea.com.

William Sonnemaker, MS, PES, CES, CSCS, is the CEO of Catalyst Fitness and an award-winning personal trainer, including IDEA's 2007 international personal trainer of the year, a National Academy of Sports Medicine 2007 Pursuit of Excellence winner, and Atlanta's Best Trainer since 2005. His many credentials include professional certifications from the American College of Sports Medicine and other top organizations, and extensive experience working with cardiac patients. His Web site is www.catalyst fitness.com.

Richard Stoltz, PhD, CAPT, USN, has been a mental health professional for over thirty years. During his twenty-two years in the Navy, he has served in numerous administrative and clinical capacities. He currently serves as the assistant chief of staff at the U.S. Navy's Bureau of Medicine and Surgery.

H. Robert Superko, MD, FACC, FAHA, FACSM, is the executive director of the Center for Genomics and Human Health at St. Joseph's Translational Research Institute in Atlanta. His background includes numerous research projects and scientific publications, directing Stanford University's Lipid Research Clinic and Laboratory, and the Cholesterol Research Center at the University of California, Berkeley. Dr. Superko wrote the book *Before the Heart Attacks* to help explain detailed aspects of heart disease risk factors that go beyond the standard risk factors. The Web site is www .HeartDisease.org.

Lisa M. Tate, as the CEO of Women Heart: The National Coalition for Women with Heart Disease, heads the only advocacy, education, and support organization in the United States dedicated solely to serving women living with heart disease. Previously, Ms. Tate was the vice president for public affairs for the National Association of Children's

Hospitals and a public affairs manager for the American Academy of Pediatrics. Her organization's Web site is www.womenheart.org.

Helen Thomas is a legendary question asker, news service reporter, columnist, and member of the White House press corps. She served for almost sixty years as a correspondent and White House bureau chief for United Press International. Ms. Thomas has covered every president since President Kennedy and was famous for challenging presidents from her front-row seat during press conferences. Ms. Thomas's Wikipedia biography is at http://en.wikipedia.org/wiki/Helen_Thomas.

Paige Waehner is a personal trainer certified through the American Council on Exercise, a freelance writer, and has more than thirteen years of exercise experience. She trains her Chicago clients in-home as well as online at Plus One Active. Ms. Waehner authored the book *About.com Guide to Getting in Shape* as well as several other books and many articles for major journals. Her Web site is http://exercise.about.com.

Kim Allan Williams, MD, FACC, is an expert in clinical and nuclear cardiology and the 2008 board chairperson for the Association of Black Cardiologists. He also serves on the Board of Trustees of the American College of Cardiology and the American Board of Internal Medicine (Cardiovascular Diseases). Dr. Williams was voted one of Chicago's top doctors in 1996, 2000, 2004, and 2007. His organization's Web site is www.uchospitals.edu.

Cary Wing, EdD, is the executive director of the Medical Fitness Association, dedicated to defining industry standards of excellence for medical fitness centers. Dr. Wing has more than twenty-five years of experience in the health and wellness field, including an advisory status with the American Council on Exercise and the American Heart Association. She gives frequent presentations on women's health issues. Her organization's Web site is www .medicalfitness.org.

Patty Wooten, RN, BSN, has more than thirty-eight years of experience in nursing, including many years as a cardiac nurse. After witnessing firsthand the power of therapeutic humor, she created an educational consulting company in Santa Cruz, California, called Jest for the Health of It. Ms. Wooten has entertained audiences around the world and is a veteran of countless radio shows, television shows, and print media, including NBC's *Real Life* and *USA Today.* Her Web site is www.jesthealth.com.

Paul Yurachek is a certified financial planner, attorney, CPA, and senior financial adviser with Gurtz, Yuracheck and Associates, a financial advisory practice of Ameriprise Financial Services in Bethesda, Maryland. Mr. Yurachek is a former employee of the Internal Revenue Service and specializes in retirement planning, tax planning, and estate planning.

Index

274 · *Index*

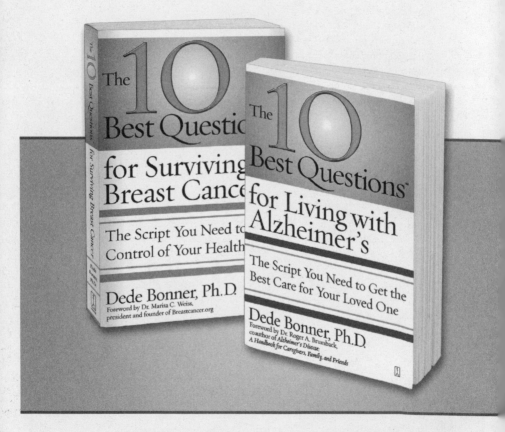
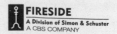